A

NON-SMOKER

AT LAST

Ambros Prechtl, ND PhD

Revised Edition

I dedicate this little book of mine to all my smoking friends, hoping to welcome them soon in the happy club of ex-smokers; to my grandchildren – Johannes und Matthias... Kelsey... John Rafael, Gabriel and Michael... Pauline, Jamilla, Jasmine and Patrick; to my kid sister Elisabeth.; to the three most important women in my life – Beate, requiescat in pace... Fe, aka Wolfie,,,; and last, but by no means least, to Elsie, my Cape Breton Rose.

CONTENTS

INTRODUCTION

There is no lack of books on how to give up smoking. I have listed six of them in the bibliography at the end of this book. All of them are available in inexpensive paperback editions. Each of them offers advice on how to become and how to remain a non-smoker; some of them expose the hazards of smoking (No.'s 3, 4 and 6 in the bibliographic list at the end); one extols the pleasures of a life without smoking (No. 4); two look at the history of smoking (No.'s 4 and 6); one reviews changing public attitudes towards smoking and moves to protect the rights of non-smokers (No.'s 4 and 6); and they call attention to the efforts of the corporate pushers of nicotine to keep old smokers hooked, to recruit new victims for the addiction and to fight the growing pressure of public hostility to smoking (No.'s 4 and 6). Why then another book about smoking?

Because all the books that have been written do not go far enough. They persist in viewing smoking as a problem in isolation, one that can be licked by any smoker who sincerely wants to quit provided he uses the right tricks and techniques. They fail to view smoking as what it really is -- a symptom of a bigger problem; namely, impaired health.

The common addictions -- to wit, the addictions to nicotine, to caffeine and to sugar -- are as much the result of impaired health as they are the cause of it. A healthy body not only does not need these substances; it rejects them. The corollary -- repair your damaged health, and the addictions will all but take care of themselves. And this is essentially the message of my book: to show the veteran smoker who has tried every other way to quit and failed how to rebuild his health and fitness so that in the end the curse of smoking will drop from him like a ripe fruit. It did for me, four decades ago, and I am doubly the winner. I am superbly fit and healthy, and I am rid of smoking.

I

BIOGRAPHY OF A SMOKER

The American Cancer Society estimates that in the decade between 1964 and 1974, when the evidence linking smoking with cancer and cardiovascular degeneration became so massive that it could not be ignored any longer, some 40 million Americans set out to give up smoking but only about one-quarter of them succeeded. These figures divided by ten would fairly represent the Canadian scene. It is this grand army of veteran smokers that this book is intended for -- the millions of men and women who would like to quit but don't know how.

I was one of them myself for 28 years. Born and raised in Germany, I started to smoke at the end of World War II, when the Americans moved in. I was all of 12 years old then. All through the war, cigarettes had been scarce in Germany, and for most of the war they had been rationed. Near the end of the war,as Germany lost its last tobacco-producing territorial possessions, cigarettes became so scarce that one could not getthem, coupons or no coupons, unless one had equally scarce commodities to trade for them -- food, coffee, clothing, car parts, etc. Many Germans grew some tobacco in their vegetable gardens, and they learned how to dry, cure and toast it themselves. Tobacco products sold in the stores, apart from being extremely scarce, were obviously adulterated by the admixture of non-tobacco varieties of the local flora; for they smelled and tasted terrible.

With the coming of the American troops, black market operations dealing in American cigarettes sprang up quickly. I got into the act with two friends of mine. German farmers were only to eager to get their hand on American cigarettes; the Americans, having lived on combat rations of dried and canned food for months, were hungry for fresh food such as eggs, meat and fruit. My friends and I became the middlemen and we quickly earned for ourselves the reputation of being honest and dependable traders. We also became the objects of envy and admiration among our peers; for we had what few Germans could boast -- genuine American cigarettes. We smoked ostentatiously and we became hooked at the ripe age of 13.

By the time I was 15, I was quite hopelessly addicted. Though I could not smoke at home -- my father, himself a heavy smoker, would have disowned me if he had known that I smoked – I managed to go through half a pack a day. After I left home to go to university, I quickly graduated to a pack a day. About that time I made my first of many futile attempts to quit. Active in sports, I hoped to improve my performance by quitting; however, after a number of failures I quit quitting, and for the next ten years I smoked, resigned that there was nothing I could do about it.

I sneered at the first reports that linked smoking with lung cancer and heart disease. But gradually I realized that, with every cigarette I smoked, I committed a bit of suicide, and I embarked on more futile attempts to free myself from the addiction. After each abortive attempt, I smoked more than before. During the last two years of my career as a smoker, I went through two to three packs a day.

I felt terrible, physically and mentally. Physically I had most of the symptoms of the veteran smoker: bad taste in my mouth all day, especially in the morning; eyes sore and blood- shot much of the time; short-windedness -- athlete that I had been once, I'd huff and puff after a brisk walk the length of two city blocks or after climbing two flights of stairs at anything but a snail's pace; con-stant cough, with violent fits of coughing in the morning. Psychologically, I was afraid of the hazards of smoking but I was even more afraid of the misery of quitting; I had developed a full-fledged inferiority complex regarding my powers of self-discipline; I felt guilty with every cigarette I smoked and my self-esteem was low, but there seemed no hope.

What I had found most demoralizing about quitting was the fact that, even after several months of not smoking, temptation did not cease. True, the urge to smoke overcame me less and less frequently, and sometimes I might not remember that there was such a thing as a cigarette for a whole day. But inevitably, sooner or later, the craving would be back. I had talked to my doctor about it. What he had to say merely deepened the despair. "You can give up smoking," he had told me, "but you cannot ever give up wanting a smoke." And an uncle of mine, who gave up smoking at the age of 52, only to start smoking again on his sixtieth birthday, used to tell me how he had made a pact with himself that, if he should live to 60, he would start to smoke again; for then life would be more or less over for him and it would not matter much if he should shorten it by smoking again. "All those eight years," he used to tell anyone willing to listen, "the craving for a smoke never left me completely; the only thing that kept me going was the cigarette I had promised myself for my sixtieth birthday." The hoplessness of it! The hopelessness of having to live with it for years, perhaps for the rest of my life.

I know better now. I know that one can give up not only smoking but also wanting to smoke. So take heart: if someone as hopelessly hooked and as totally demoralized as I was could get himself unhooked, there is more than just hope for you. You need two things to quit. One of them you already have – a genuine desire to quit; the other is something this book will give you -- a better understanding of the hold smoking has on you and of the means to break that hold.

II

THE HOLD SMOKING HAS ON YOU

In the chapter "Why You Really Smoke," Mr. Brean discusses at some length the reasons why people start to smoke, get hooked and continue to smoke though they would very much like to quit. (How to Stop Smoking, pp. 45 - 48) It is interesting to read what Mr. Brean has to say there, especially about the pleasure of smoking. As he puts it,

> "Only the naive say they smoke for pleasure. Usually the veteran smoker is more bitterly honest."

The veteran smoker knows indeed that he smokes, less because smoking gives him pleasure, than because he is so dependent on smoking that he experiences withdrawal symptoms after only short periods without it, and he needs to smoke to "cure" the discomfort of these withdrawal symptoms.

Let us look more closely at this dependence on smoking. When reduced to its simplest terms, it turns out to have two components -- a stimulative one and a sedative one. When a smoker lights a cigarette, certain chemicals in the smoke, chief among them nicotine, cause the release of adrenalin into his bloodstream and he experiences a "lift." But soon afterwards, another set of chemicals begins to slow the flow of his blood by constricting his blood vessels. His whole body shifts into a lower metabolic gear and he "calms down."

Now, a healthy body does not need either the stimulative or the sedative effect of smoking. A dependence on one or the other is a sign of impaired health. To be more specific, a dependence on the stimulative effect is a fairly certain sign that the body's energy-producing systems do not function effectively; a dependence on the sedative effect is a sign that the ictim's nerves are in bad shape. The veteran smoker who hopes to become a non-smoker at last must remedy these conditions so as to break the physiological hold smoking has on him.

Fortunately, he need not be a nutritional or medical expert to do so. His own body, best of nutritional medics, will do it for him if only he provides the right conditions for it to function in. Just what these conditions are will be explained in Chapter IV. There is, however, one biochemical process which he should understand in some detail -- his body's sugar metabolism. At the very least he should know how to avoid disturbing it unnecessarily; for, a disturbed sugar metabolism can make the job of giving up smoking very difficult, if not impossible.

For one's body and mind to function well, one's blood sugar must remain within certain limits. Either too much of it or too little results in sensations of discomfort and in the disturbance of certain vital physiological processes. Of course some fluctuations are inevitable. After a meal, the blood sugar rises; but, before it can go too high, insulin is released to make it go down until it reaches its normal lower limit. Now, if the insulin-producing mechanism is faulty, one of two things happens: if too little insulin enters the blood, diabetes results; if too much is released, the result is low blood sugar or hypoglycemia.

Among the first sensations to be felt when the blood sugar level drops below what is normal for a given individual are intense hunger, punctuated frequently by hunger pains in the pit of the stomach and occasionally by hunger headaches, a general feeling of weakness, drowsiness and irritability. A further drop may lead to severe nervousness, anxiety, cold sweats, forgetfulness, etc. If blood sugar levels drop dangerously low, the results may be mental confusion, depression, unnaturally rapid heart beat, crying spells, general lack of coordination and finally unconsciousness.

Blood sugar plays a part in the transport of oxygen to the cells. If there is not enough glucose in the blood, too little oxygen reaches the cells. As a result, muscles feel weak and the nervous system cannot function properly. The effects of oxygen starvation due to low blood sugar are much the same as those of oxygen starvation due to external conditions such as drowning or complications of childbirth. If the external condition is not corrected in time, the brain may be damaged beyond repair though the victim may live. Severe hypoglycemia, too, if not remedied in time, can result in brain damage.

In the present context we are less concerned with hypoglycemia so severe as to cause brain damage than with lesser, more every-day manifestations of it, which it is nevertheless very important to bring under control for anyone who hopes to quit smoking. For, hypoglycemia even in its milder forms upsets the body's sense of well-being and disturbs its ability to function efficiently. The body tries to remedy the condition by craving things which have brought relief in the past; and, the more severe the drop of the blood sugar level, the more irresistible the cravings.

Among the things which can bring relief from the pangs of hypoglycemia are coffee, sugar and nicotine. Sugar brings relief directly. Closely related to glucose (blood sugar) in its chemical make-up, it is easily and quickly converted to glucose in the digestive tract and absorbed as such into the blood stream. Coffee -- tea too, for that matter -- and nicotine bring relief in a more indirect way. They stimulate the adrenal glands to release adrenalin. Adrenalin, in turn, causes the liver to convert some of its stored glycogen into glucose and to discharge it into the blood. In either case, up goes the blood sugar level, the sensations of discomfort subside and the crisis is over for the time being.

But the relief is short-lived. Let's see what happens if the victim of hypoglycemia eats a chocolate bar. The refined sugar of the bar is quickly converted to glucose and absorbed into the blood. He experiences almost instant relief from the sensations of discomfort associated with hypoglycemia. However, the internal backlash is quick and inexorable: too much glucose enters the blood too fast and the pancreas, whose duty it is to keep the blood sugar level from soaring too high, panics and releases more insulin than necessary. In consequence, the blood level of glucose drops lower than it should be, the sensations of discomfort return and so does the craving for another chocolate bar.

One person's chocolate bar is another person's cup of coffee or tea or a CIGARETTE. For some people it is all of them. From past experience, the body "remembers" what substances bring relief, and it clamors for them as soon as it feels the firs pinches of hypoglycemia. The more severe the drop in blood sugar, the more over-powering the craving for something that promises relief. How ironic that people going through the misery of nicotine withdrawal should "spoil" themselves with cup after cup of coffee and/or candy! For both coffee and sugar produce, after an initial rise of the blood sugar level, the inevitable drop of it, which intensifies the budding non-smoker's craving for a cigarette.

What then can you do to bring the fluctuations of blood sugar under control? The answer is really quite simple: 1. Adjust your eating habits -- instead of three square meals a day, have five or six small ones; 2. Avoid the substances which unbalance your sugar metabolism -- sugar, and in fact all other refined carbohydrates; coffee and tea; soft drinks; and nicotine. Sound like a tall order? It isn't really. Just do it and you will be surprised how naturally one thing will lead to the next. Start out by eliminating the substance you find easiest to do without and gradually work your way up to the most difficult one; to wit, nicotine. By the time you get to the last and most difficult one, your sugar metabolism will be so well balanced that eliminating nicotine from the routine of your existence will be, if not downright easy, at least possible, though you be one of the most hopelessly hooked smokers.

You may wonder why five or six small meals a day instead of the customary three square meals. It takes an overactive pancreas some time to calm down. Till it has calmed down, it may cause sporadic drops of blood sugar by discharging insulin at the least provocation or when there is no apparent provocation at all. A steady supply of blood sugar from frequent small meals compensates for these sporadic drops.

You must also be curious what foods you can eat in place of the ones you have been told to avoid. Use freely all unrefined carbohydrates such as whole-wheat products, whole rolled oats, brown (unpolished) rice, potatoes baked in their skins, etc. Fresh vegetables and fruit are a must. But go easy on the very sweet dried fruit such as raisins, figs and dates, at least until you are sure your blood sugar metabolism has settled down. And go easy on fruit juices -- not more than two or three ounces at a time, preferably diluted with a little water – for they supply too much sugar too fast. Finally, you should lean heavily on the protein foods such as eggs, fish, fowl, cheese, plain yogurt, milk and -- in moderation -- meat. Protein foods are the ones that "stick to your ribs." They digest slowly, and though they are partly converted to glucose, this happens so slowly that there is no risk of flooding the blood with glucose which might spook the pancreas into a fit of hyperactivity.

You will find more detailed information on what to

eat in Chapter IV. Ideally you should read one of the books on hypoglycemia listed in the bibliography and adopt the dietary approach it recommends. The well-known Atkins diet also helps to bring an errant blood sugar under control. Finally, there is a ready-made diet plan tailored for the needs of the hypoglycemic -- that of Weight Watchers of America. It bans all refined carbohydrates and it insists on frequent small meals. No wonder that people who adopt it not only lose weight but discover that suddenly they can do what they have tried to do without success in the past -- give up smoking.

III

SOME MISCONCEPTIONS
ABOUT QUITTING

One very common misconception about quitting has already been dealt with -- the notion that, though one may give up smoking, one cannot give up wanting a smoke. There are several more to be cleared up. They can cause much unnecessary anguish to the potential quitter who accepts them as though they were true.

One of them is the fear that giving up smoking inevitably means putting on weight. Unfortunately this is what happens to many people when they quit because they go about it the wrong way; i.e., they replace cigarettes with junk foods of the worst kind such as candy, sweet pastry, ice-cream, etc. To the uninformed this may seem a perfectly innocent and legitimate reward for giving up smoking. The bitter truth of it, however, is that the ex-smoker who spoils himself with sugar junk is in for double trouble: on one hand, sugar junking will perpetuate his hypoglycemia, the very condition which is at the bottom of the craving for nicotine; on the other hand, sugar junking will make him gain weight. But it need not happen to you. If you follow the procedure for stabilizing your sugar metabolism set out in Chapter II and adopt the strategies discussed in Chapter IV, you will get by very well without sugar junk, and you will not gain weight. In fact, if you are heavier than you would like to be, you can look forward to losing some unwanted pounds even while you get yourself unhooked from nicotine. So, no more of the fallacious logic that rationalizes: Thin is beautiful. Smoking keeps me thin. Therefore smoking keeps me beautiful.

Another misconception about quitting is the notion

that giving up smoking is largely a matter of willpower. I used to subscribe to this notion myself. Before every new attempt to quit, I would muster all I had of willpower, hoping against hope to ride to victory on the sheer strength of it. And invariably I failed, and I continued to fail till I understood that willpower isn't just some metaphysical entity, independent of the body, of which some lucky people have much and some unlucky people (myself included) have little.

Whatever we may call the whole of which willpower is a part -- mind, mental make-up, moral nature -- that whole is itself not something which exists in isolation but a function of the nervous system. Anything that alters significantly the chemistry of the nervous system affects mind in general and will power in particular. We readily concede that medical drugs can do this. People on certain medications such as antihistamines or some of the major tranquilizers are warned not to drive while under the influence of their medications. We don't know enough about hypoglycemia to issue similar warnings to people suffering from it. And we still believe that the coffee addict, the sugar junkie and the smokers who cannot liberate themselves from their addictions merely lack willpower instead of according them the extenuating circumstances we so readily accord to people on certain mind-altering medications. And the addicts themselves, by subscribing to the misconception, make things unnecessarily difficult for themselves when they set out to quit.

It is of crucial importance for the smoker who hopes to quit to understand that hypoglycemia has adverse effects on the chemistry of the nervous system. One of these effects is that it erodes that mythical entity which we call willpower. When your blood sugar is up to par, it is easy to display great strength of willpower: you can disdainfully walk past the display window of the pastry shop; you can smugly say "No, thank you" when a falsely compassionate smoker offers you a cigarette. But let your blood sugar drop, let the sensations of discomfort begin to pinch you and let the craving stir in every cell of your being -- how quickly all your strength of willpower can vanish into thin air!

To make matters worse, this erosion of will power is accompanied by other "mental changes." A friend of mine, who when in his "right mind" frowns on jogging, has confessed to me that on occasion hypoglycemia so altered his views that he himself broke into a trot to get to the pastry shop a little faster. Every veteran smoker knows how rational thinking wanes when the craving waxes. The other day a smoker told me that once he walked three miles in a snowstorm to get his hands on a pack of cigarettes. Another smoker admitted that he had a taxi bring him a pack in the middle of the night, at a total cost several times the value of the pack of cigarettes.

So, be wise smoker: if you hope to quit, don't place your bets on willpower. You are better off to place your bets on correcting your body chemistry -- stabilizing your sugar metabolism, above all. Doing that you keep your willpower strong and you take the wind out of temptation's sails.

Another misconception about quitting, perhaps the most insidious one of them all, is really less a misconception than a half-conception. It is the notion that the smoker should quit because smoking is bad for his health. Now, while there is nothing wrong with this notion itself, it is nevertheless only one side of the coin. The other ide of it -- commonly ignored but, if anything, more important for the would-be quitter -- bears the message that the addiction to nicotine, like the addictions to caffeine and sugar, is a result, not the cause of impaired health.

The significance of this message for the veteran of many futile attempts to quit can hardly be overstated. It shows the problem of quitting in an entirely new light: instead of being itself the ill to be combatted, smoking turns out to be a symptom of a larger ill -- impaired health; and, to deal effectively with the symptom, it is necessary to deal first with the underlying cause. In other words, to get himself unhooked, the veteran smoker must first repair his health; for in repairing his health, he will so lessen his dependence on nicotine that giving up smoking will become, if not exactly easy, at least manageable.

The perfectly healthy body does not need the stimulants of caffeine, sugar or nicotine; on the contrary, it rejects them. A healthy youngster, who explores the doubtful pleasures of smoking for the first time, may end up experiencing most unpleasant sensations as his body, in protest against the hygienic insult, threatens to eject as much of the offending substance as possible in both directions at once. Perhaps you remember yourself how violently your body reacted the first time you inflicted nicotine on it. If you had "listened" to your body then, you would not have got hooked on nicotine.

Understanding this basic truth takes much of the mystery out of the question why, given the same circumstances, some people become addicts while others don't. Think of two people smoking for the first time. One is in an excellent state of health; the energy control systems of his body are perfectly tuned. He not only gets no "lift" from the nicotine; he ends up feeling sick. The other person, his energy systems badly out of tune, does experience a real lift. When the two confront nicotine again, the first one is more likely than not to feel an aversion to it while the second one is likely "to feel like a smoke again." And smoking will worsen the condition which predisposes the potential addict to become a real addict in the first place. Similarly, the other addictive substances -- caffeine and sugar -- pose little temptation for a genuinely healthy person because they do nothing for him; but they constitute a very real temptation for him whose energy control systems are out of tune. The moral of it is obvious: if a healthy body rejects nicotine or at least does not need it, the smoker who hopes to quit can best prepare himself for the impending battle by rebuilding his health.

Let's take stock. It is possible then not merely to give up smoking but also to overcome the desire to smoke completely. Moreover, giving up smoking need not result in a weight gain. Further, if you have doubts about your willpower, get your sugar metabolism back in tune. Finally, the best preparation for the fight against nicotine is a program of rebuilding health.

IV

SIX STRATEGIES TO GET YOU READY

For decades, big business has spent vast sums of money on advertizing designed to condition us to believe in and to expect the instant magic solution to all our problems, with little effort -- if any -- of our own. Over-weight? Why, your friendly druggist has the answer – an instamagic reducing pill or an instamagic reducing formula of a liquid protein diet. No need to change a lifestyle which is the real cause of the weight problem. No need to suffer. Constipation? All you need is one of scores of instamagic laxatives for sale at your friendly neighborhood drugstore. Feel unglamorous, unbeautiful, unsuccessful, left out? Why, start smoking the cigarette which beautiful people smoke under palm trees, and you will feel beautiful too.... Worried about what smoking may do to your lungs? Stop worrying. The mago-scientists have found a way to filter all the harmfulness out of smoking. If you put their instamagic filter between your cigarette and your lungs, you can have your pleasure without the risk.... And, should you wish to give up smoking altogether, those same mago-scientists offer you a pill which instantly turns the most inveterate smoker against smoking....

Of course the instant magic does not work. The weight watcher regains the pounds lost thanks to the instamagic reducing pill faster than (s)he took them off. The instamagic anti-smoke pill neither corrects the biochemical imbalances, which are largely responsible for the nicotine addiction, nor eliminates the craving for a cigarette. The smoker who invests money and hope in it goes on craving his nicotine fix; the only thing different for him is that, if he smokes while the effect of the pill lasts, he will get sick. However, the fear of getting sick adds another stress to an already stressful situation and sooner or later he will quit the pill to resume smoking without fear.

There is no instamagic shortcut to getting yourself ready for quitting. To get there, you must invest some time and effort in a number of a preparatory strategies. If you do, you will in time be ready to do battle and you will come away a winner. Think of it -- you a non-smoker at last! If you don't get yourself ready, you are not unlike a man who, having lived through a debilitating illness, decides to embark on an arduous journey without waiting for his body to regain its strength first. Chances are that he will not get there at all; but, even if he does, he gains nothing by making the journey more troublesome than it need be.

Below, several major preparatory strategies will be discussed. You will be given enough information about each one to understand what part it plays in the program of getting you ready and how to go about practicing it. However, if at all possible, you should do a little extra reading about them; for, the better informed you are, the more you will be convinced of their value and the more conscientiously you will practice them.   For suggestions of further reading, turn to the bibliography at the end of this book.

We, the citizens of the 2nd decade of the 21st century, know so much about so many things but so little about our own bodies. We know about the latest stock market trends; the media keep us posted on the latest developments in Russia and on the death toll of the latest earthquake in the Far East; we are familiar with the surface of the moon and the floor of the oceans; most of us know a great deal about the automobiles we drive, the machines we use in our homes and in our offices; before we use a new piece of equipment, whether it is a pocket calculator or a computer, we usually take the trouble to read the operating instructions. But we are deplorably ignorant about our own bodies, the most important and the most complex of all the pieces of machinery, which we use every day of our lives. What we do get of operating instructions concerning our bodies is often mis-leading, sometimes downright fraudulent and   harmful: we are told that we are sure to start our day radiant with energy if we have a certain sugar-polluted cereal for breakfast; we are led to believe that a chocolate bar is a good source of energy; cosmetics companies misinform us that it is good for our armpits to be serviced with antiperspirants. Daily, hourly we are deluged with this sort of misinformation, but few of us have any genuine knowledge of the real needs of our bodies. That we leave to the experts -- the doctor, the nutritionist, the track coach.

But we cannot surrender the responsibility for our health to others with impunity, not even to our family doctor. No one, not even our doctor, can do for us what is necessary to build and to maintain health. Only we ourselves can. Our doctor cannot steer us past the candy counter or the pastry shop; he cannot abstain from sugar or caffeine for us; he cannot do that daily minimum of exercise for us which is a must if we are to stay or to be-come healthy; he cannot quit smoking for us. The best of our doctors -- those who are concerned more with the prevention of disease than with the treatment of symptoms -- would have us well informed, but they do not have the time to inform us. We must do that ourselves. The worst of our doctors would rather have us ignorant: for the less we know, the less likely we are to question anything they do to us and the more dependent we are on their services.

Get yourself started then on a program of self-education in matters of fitness and health. Anyone should do this, not only the smoker who hopes to quit. Keep at it at least till you have yourself unhooked from smoking. Of course, if you know what's good for you, you will keep at it long after you have become a non-smoker.

Let's have a look now at the major strategies which you are to adopt and to practice to get yourself ready for quitting.

1. Eat yourself (back) into good health;
2. Abstain from caffeine, sugar and things that contain a lot of sugar such as soft drinks and pastry;
3. Treat yourself to an occasional fast;
4. Exercise;
5. Learn to relax through yoga and meditation;
6. Practice the technique of auto-suggestion.

As much as possible, practice all these strategies. Start with the ones you find easiest and gradually work your way up to the ones you find hardest. Since each strategy contributes its part towards improving your fitness and your health, each successive step will be easier to adopt. Giving up smoking is essentially just another strategy in a general program of rebuilding health; but, because it is the most difficult one, at least for the heavy smoker, it will be left to the end, in the hope that by the time you get to it, you will be in such fine shape that your body can get on very well without nicotine and quitting will be easy.

If there is among the strategies one which you cannot or do not want to practice, do not despair. Like most things human, this program of getting you ready is not an all-or-nothing proposition; it is rather one of more or less. The more of the strategies you practice, the more vigorously ready you will be to quit when the time comes. Yet, if you should enter the final battle having practiced only two or three of the strategies, you would still be incomparably better off than you would be if you went into it cold. Without knowing it, some people may be so nearly ready that it will take only one or two of the strategies to get them over the hump. Perhaps that's why some people who have tried and failed before suddenly manage to quit after they have jogged for a few months or practiced yoga or meditated.   Perhaps that's why someone, having declared in a sudden fit of anger that he is going to quit, may actually stick with it. Of course it is not the anger that carries him to success; the anger is merely an occasion for a readiness already there to manifest itself.

One more thing. Don't lose sight of the fact that your main objective is to free yourself from the curse of smoking. Once you are safely a non-smoker, you may ease up on some of the strategies or drop them altogether if you find them annoying.   The practice of autosuggestion, for instance, you may discontinue altogether. You may permit yourself a cup of coffee now and then or a cup of tea. But don't overdo it.   Coffee and tea are not substances that are necessary for good health.

Major strategy 1: Eat yourself (back) into good health. Except in exceptional cases, good health is not a matter of accident; it is not something which capricious gods bestow on some and withhold from others; it is not the gift of doctors: it is your own responsibility, yours to make or to mar. I have heard it said that sanity is merely the kind of madness that is prevalent. Nowhere is this truer than in matters of health and nutrition. The few who take the responsibility of looking after their health seriously are decried as mad; the many who act as though it were their appointed task to destroy their health are considered sane -- those who eat junk, drink coffee and soft drinks from dawn to dusk, smoke and grow fat from lack of exercise.

Our bodies are marvelous pieces of biological engineering. They have the wisdom to build themselves, the wisdom to maintain themselves and -- if given half a chance -- the wisdom to repair themselves. If you are sick, no doctor can cure you. Your body must do the curing. The best a good doctor can do is to assist your body in curing itself. Nevertheless, as one wag put it, "My body, with God's help, cures itself, but my doctor takes the fee." Well, it is reassuring to know that you have at your service at all times the best of physicians – your own body. And, if you make the major strategies discussed in this chapter part of your daily routine, you will go a long way towards providing this best of physicians with the biological environment it needs to rebuild optimal health for you.

Proper nutrition is probably the most important one of these strategies. You may think food is food. You may think that there is no significant difference other than taste between natural foods on one hand and highly processed and refined food on the other hand. But your body won't be fooled. If you prefer easy convenience foods to foods which you have to prepare yourself, you pay a doubly steep price -- immediately, in terms of dollars and cents, for the food processor makes you pay for his labor of corrupting your food; and later, in terms of lost health.

It is amazing how little the majority of people know about nutrition. It is equally amazing how much, thanks to advertizing, people know about nutrition that is wrong and harmful. Take only that most pernicious and ubiquitous piece of misinformation that we need sugar for energy. Here the advertizing magician in the pay of the sugar growers deliberately packs two terms into one as though they were one and the same thing -- sugar and blood sugar -- in order to confuse and to mislead. For, while it is true that the level of one's energy rises and falls with the concentration of glucose in one's blood, it is equally true that putting sugar into your stomach is a quick and sure way of unbalancing your blood levels of glucose; and it makes no difference whether the sugar comes from the sugar bowl, from ice-cream, from pastry or from candy. Remember what I told you above about eating a chocolate bar. Sugar therefore is not a good source of energy. Similar nutritional misinfor-mation abounds about other highly processed and/or refined food: a great many supermarket shoppers believe that white bread is good for them because it has been enriched or that margarine is preferable to genuine butter. How long before they will believe that synthetic coffee cream is better than milk or that imitation egg is better than real egg.

My dietary suggestions will necessarily be sketchy and incomplete. They will probably raise as many questions as they answer. For instance, when I tell you that you should not drink while you eat, not even water, or that you should get a tablespoon of cold-pressed oil a day, you will surely wonder why. If you are really interested, you can find the answers in the books listed under nutrition in the bibliography. As I have suggested before, you should really launch on a program of nutritional self-education. At the very least, you should read one or two of the books on nutrition in the bibliography. However, if you cannot or will not do either, the suggestions I offer, below and in Appendix A, will at least get you started in the right direction.

Here are a few general cautions, which it would be well for everyone to heed, not only for those who hope to quit smoking:

1.   Avoid foods that do not spoil. If a food does not

spoil, it is probably so full of chemicals or so empty of nutrients that even spoilage bacteria stay away from it. Eat only food that spoils, but eat it before it spoils.

2.   Avoid coffee and tea, at least till you have quit smoking.

3.   Avoid sugar and white flour and all foods that contain them. No candy, no cookies, no cakes; no ice-cream, none of the commercial flavored yogurts. If you want a sweet treat turn to fruit. Mash a ripe banana and stir it into a bit of unflavored, unsweetened yogurt. Delicious!

4.   Avoid foods that contain chemical additives.

5.   Avoid unconditionally the pure junk foods like soft drinks, potato chips and other party foods such as soda crackers, pretzels, etc. These substances give you next to nothing of nutritional value -- virtually no vitamins, no minerals, no fiber; very little, if any, protein. But they give you lots of empty calories -- the last thing most of us need – and undesirable additives.

6.   Avoid commercial sauces and salad dressings. Most of them contain sugar and chemical additives.

7.   Go easy on the salt shaker. If most of your food is unprocessed and unrefined, you get nearly all the salt you need from it.

8.   Don't consider milk a drink: consider it a food. Have a glass of milk between meals for a snack, but do not drink milk with your meals.

9.   Don't drink with your meals at all. Drink up to half anour before a meal and don't drink again till at least an hour afterwards.

10. You cannot hope to build health or to maintain it on a diet of fast foods. When in doubt, skip a meal. Rather than inflict a doughnut and coffee on your organism, wait till you can get at real food -- food that has been processed only as much as is necessary to make it eatable. And remember, the more of your food you eat raw, the better it is for you and the less energy and time it

takes to prepare it.

The intent of the nutritional program is that you should eat yourself into a state of health so nearly perfect that, as much as that is possible, all hidden hungers resulting from nutritional deficiencies will be stilled and biochemical imbalances will be corrected. For, most nutritional deficiencies and most biochemical imbalances can translate themselves into cravings, which in turn can add to the difficulties of the ex-smoker during and after the withdrawal period.

Remember, all your food should be eaten in as natural and unaltered a state as possible. Even cooking, the least noxious form of processing, destroys some nutrients, above all the al-important enzymes. Therefore you should eat raw some food that you can eat raw every day. I eat virtually all my food raw, even meat. I "cure" it the way Italians cure meat for salami or for prociutto and then chase it through my meat grinder to produce delisious raw, cured ground meat. Besides, if your diet consists largely of natural and unaltered food, you need not worry whether you get the right amounts of each of the three main components of food -- carbohydrates, fats and proteins. Of the first two you are more likely to get too much than too little. As for protein, even if you avoid meat altogether, you are not likely to become protein deficient unless you are one of the vegans, that minority among vegetarians who refuse to eat any animal product at all, even eggs, cheese, or milk. For, most unrefined foods contain some protein, even fruit and vegetables; and such a humble food as rolled oats -- unrefined, non-instant, if you know what's good for you -- is an excel-lent source of high-quality protein, even before milk has been added. No need to waste time and energy cooking it either. Just pour hot milk over it and let it sit for a few minutes. Then add your favorite flavoring agent -- a few drops of vanilla, a mashed banana, a teaspoon of black-strap molasses, and you end up with a delicious and nutritious breakfast. It is people whose caloric needs are met largely from junk foods that should be worried about their protein intake.

I am going to pause here in my nutritional lecture because I want you to get on with the job of finding out about the rest of the major strategies. For more detailed information about what you should eat, turn to Appendix A. You will also find some suggestions regarding vitamin and mineral supplements there.

Major strategy 2: Abstain from coffee and tea, at least while you are trying to quit; from sugar and soft drinks, especially the caffeinated ones, till the end of your time. Even though I have already sounded several warnings against these substances, I feel they deserve more attention. But let me reassure you first that, though I feel strongly that you would be better off if you bade them farewell permanently, I am not about to pronounce a permanent ban on them. What I suggest is that you should abstain from them for some time before you quit smoking and for some time afterwards. Once you are safely established as a non-smoker -- Just think of it, you a NON-SMOKER! -- you may go back to having an occasional cup of coffee or tea, maybe even a candy bar. Remember, the one thing you want to quit for good is smoking. Giving up coffee, tea, even candy, for a time will help you to get there. Surely that's worth the brief sacrifice. But you should not try to give up coffee, tea, candy and smoking all at the same time. That would be asking the impossible of yourself. And that's why I suggest that you wean yourself from these substances some time before you quit smoking.

There is another reason why the new ex-smoker should avoid these two substances as much as possible until he is sure that he will remain an ex-smoker -- the fact that the two substances trigger the urge to smoke by association. For years, a coffee and a smoke or a tea and a smoke have been linked together so inseparably in his association pattern that either one has come to bring in its wake a need for the other: he has a cup of coffee, especially that first one in the morning, and he wants a smoke; he has a smoke and he wants a cup of coffee or tea.

All too many people assume that, because the substances I have been talking about -- coffee, tea and sugar -- produce no immediately apparent destructive effects, they are not harmful. The assumption is deadly wrong. True, having a cup of coffee or tea and a dough-nut is not a sudden-death affair. Neither is having a cigarette, for that matter. But all these substances are harmful if one indulges in them regularly. These are the very substances which people use to console themselves and to pamper themselves with while they go through the worst of the withdrawal misery; but in very insidious ways, these substances make the job of quitting more difficult than it need be.

All of them are guilty of robbing the body of certain nutrients. To process any food, the body needs certain vitamins and minerals. Whole, natural foods come well stocked with them; in fact, they carry more of them than is needed for their own processing, and what's left after they have been processed is credited to the body's nutritional bank account. Now sugar, coffee and tea do not supply any vitamins or minerals. To process them, the body must draw on its own reserves of nutri-ents. In other words, our three offenders rob the body of vitamins and minerals instead of supplying them. Thus sugar robs the body of B-vitamins and of various mi-nerals, among them calcium, magnesium, potassium and the trace mineral chromium. Every cup of coffee or tea you drink costs you in terms of the B-vitamins. But an adequate supply of all these substances is necessary for the proper functioning of the nervous system. Among the first symptoms to result from a deficiency of calcium or magnesium and of practically every one of the B-vitamins are nervousness, irritability, restlessness -- the very things that plague the man or woman who tries to give up smoking. Therefore abstain from these noxious substances, at least while you are getting ready to quit, so as to give your nervous system a chance to repair itself. You can aid the process by eating of the B-rich foods discussed in Appendix A.

Perhaps the most important reason why he who hopes to give up smoking should abstain from coffee, tea and sugar is that they all play a part in unbalancing the body's sugar metabolism. This in turn can make the job of quitting more difficult.

Major strategy 3: treat yourself to an occasional fast. Now, don't panic. I am not going to tell you that you cannot give up smoking unless you fast. I am simply going to tell you that fasting makes it easier to give up smoking. Read what I have to say and decide for yourself whether you want to try a 24-hour or a 48-hour fast some time soon. If not, nothing is lost.

Fasting is at least as old as man's recorded history. For thousands of years it has played a part both in religious ritual and as a technique of healing. As a technique of healing it is still widely practiced in many parts of the world. It is only in North America, really, that the majority of medical men pooh-pooh it as dangerous faddism. But even in North America there are some doctors who endorse it. One of them is Doctor Allan Cott, a New York psychiatrist of international renown. He recommends fasting unreservedly as the ultimate therapy for many of man's ills. His two books on fasting (see bibliography) are both informative and interesting.

There are various kinds of fasts. There is the absolute fast -- no food of any kind, no water. This is the fast practiced by Muslims the world over for one whole month every year. And there are modified fasts -- no food for a certain length of time but water, no food except fruit juices and water, no food except fresh, raw fruit and/or vegetables and water. Which type of fast you choose depends on what you want to accomplish. The kind of fast most commonly recommended for therapeutic purposes -- the kind Dr. Cott deals with in his two books -- means total abstention from food, solid or liquid, for a certain number of days, but liberal consumption of water; in fact, water should be drunk generously on this type of fast. "Days" here means periods of twenty-four hours, not just the hours of daylight. In this context, a one-week fast means no food at all for one week, neither during the hours of daylight nor at night. I have fasted for four to seven days more than once and felt good all the way.

The idea of going without food for more than a few hours frightens many people in North America and Europe. All too many of them believe that, if they did not have their three square meals a day, they would feel weak and could not do their work efficiently, if at all. But from volumes and volumes of literature, old and new, that have been written about fasting, it is evident that fasting is perfectly safe for most people, and that all but a very few can fast safely for several weeks and come away from the fast healthier and more energetic than they were before it. However, no layman should undertake a "therapeutic" fast of more than two or three days' duration without the supervision of a doctor who is competent in monitoring a prolonged fast. And no one should undertake even a short "therapeutic" fast without informing himself first about fasting itself and about the right way to break a fast. Someone who has fasted for say seven days -- that is, has not eaten any food at all for seven days -- can do himself harm if he does not break his fast the right way.

Seven days without food is by no means the limit. I remember the story of a small plane carrying its pilot and a passenger that crash-landed somewhere in northern Canada a few years ago. The two survived the crash-landing and until they were found, a month later, they lived on nothing but water -- water obtained from the snow they had landed in. The doctors who examined them were amazed at their good state of general health. Some Irish hunger strikers have gone without food for three months. The Guiness Book of World Records carries the story of a man who, under medical super-vision, fasted for more than a year. The purpose of his fast was to shed several hundred of the six hundred or so pounds of overweight he was carrying.

Generally speaking, a therapeutic fast -- even the short fast of one or two days, which you may undertake on your own – leaves the body-mind ensemble healthier and better able to cope with the stresses of living. Some of the more specific benefits of the therapeutic fast are:

1. A loss of weight.
2. A saving of energy. The digestion of food requires a lot pf energy. After a big meal one may feel so drowsy as to fall asleep. Not having to digest food, the body saves much energy, which can be put to use elsewhere. So, far from weakening you, fasting leaves you more energetic. Many long-distance runners of international caliber pre-pare themselves for major races by fasting for a day or two.. Some of the very best enter the marathon, that most gruelling of all running events, after a fast of one or more days; and, though they do not eat at all before the race, they do not falter with weakness.
3. A biological house cleaning. Waste matter accumulates in the body from various sources -- the

regular processing of food, the break-down of tissues through normal wear and tear, the inundation of our bodies' ecology by toxic substances from polluted food, water and air. Not having to cope with the processing of food and not having to clean up the mess that results from it, the body can get to work ridding itself of waste matter which it is normally too busy to attend to.

4. A general overhaul. Contantly the body has to repair cells that break down or are destroyed by accidental injury. Frequently it is kept so busy processing unne-cessarily big quantities of food and dealing with the poisons of junk food and nicotine that it can look after only the most pressing repairs. A fast gives it a chance to catch up on overdue chores of maintenance. And, inter-estingly, during a fast, when the body gets no building materials from food, it uses re-cycled materials -- tissues worn out or diseased that have to be taken down.

For the smoker about to quit, fasting offers another benefit: the most efficient way of eliminating accumu-lations of toxic waste, it is also the fastest way of over-coming the misery of nicotine withdrawal. Dr. Cott reports that fasting alone has made it possible for many a veteran smoker to quit (Fasting as a Way of Life, pp. 7 to 9).

Even one fast is enough to convince the novice that it is worthwhile to fast. You, too, owe it to yourself to read up on the benefits of fasting and to try at least one 24-hour "therapeutic" fast; for, the way you feel after even so short a fast will do more than anything I can say to prove to you that fasting makes sense. However, if you decide that "therapeutic" fasting is not for you, you will not seriously lower your chances of winning your fight against nicotine. I have included fasting in my list of major strategies because I think the list would be incomplete without it, not because I think that quitting is not possible without fasting.

Major strategy 4: Exercise. Everyone needs exercise, not only the man or woman who intends to give up smoking, a fact which more and more people are beginning to understand. Even some of our doctors have started seriously to counsel their patients to exercise. Nevertheless, most North Americans, young or old, and a great many Europeans still exercise very little, if at all. The trouble is that those who have the power and the money to shape public attitudes are more interested in profits than in general fitness and health. If they were genuinely interested in the latter, they could, in a matter of a few years, persuade people to accept fitness as a desirable ideal as surely as they have managed to condition millions of people to believe the pernicious piece of disinformation that one needs sugar for energy. True, our Canadian government has made some moves in the right direction. Through "participaction" it has been trying to encourage people to exercise. It has also done much to discourage smoking. More about that later. But the government's efforts to steer people towards fitness and health are largely negated by the more massive efforts of the corporate establishment to keep people hooked on denatured foods such as soft drinks and sugar junk and on cigarettes, and keeping them glued to their TV sets every moment of their free time.

As with the other major strategies, I recommend that the reader inform himself about exercise -- learn why a certain minimum of exercise is essential for fitness and health; learn how exercise is necessary to build or to maintain fitness and health; learn what, apart from building fitness, exercise can do for the man or the woman who wants to quit smoking. Probably the best book to start with is Dr. Cooper's Aerobics.

The term exercise covers a lot of ground. It includes weight-lifting and yoga, calisthenics and running, walking, swimming and many other things. While every form of exercise has something to recommend it to some people, not every form of exercise is good for everybody. However, one thing is safe to say -- for most people, any exercise at all is better than no exercise.

One of the sine-qua-non's of fitness and health is an efficient cardiovascular system, which is capable of supplying optimally all parts of the body with the necessary nutrients and building materials. And there is only one thing that can get or keep your cardiovascular system in good shape – aerobic exercise.

Aerobic exercise is exercise which makes your heart beat fast and which makes you breathe hard and sweat. The kinds of exercise that accomplish this are those which involve more or less vigorous movement of the whole body, or large parts of it, continuously for a certain length of time. Such forms of exercise as calisthenics, weight-lifting, push-ups, stretching exercises and the whole range of yoga movements and postures do not qualify as aerobic because they do not represent a sustained continuous effort. Here are some forms of exercise that do: walking, jogging, stationary running, swimming, bicycling, cross-country skiing, rowing and many games such as soccer, basketball,hockey, squash, tennis, etc.

The most important health benefit of aerobic exercise is that it reconditions your heart. A more efficient heart means more efficient transportation of nutrients to and removal of waste from all parts of the body. As your heart's efficiency increases, you will notice a gradual slowing of its beat. A slowing by about ten beats a minute in the course of a few months is not uncommon. You can check your heartbeat by checking your pulse. The slowing of your heart's beat is a good sign; it is an external manifestation of its greater efficiency, the fact that it can accomplish with fewer beats the job of sending the blood to the most distant parts of your body. That means less wear and tear for your heart and probably a greater life expectancy for you. Another important benefit of aerobic exercise is the fact that it makes you sweat; for sweating assists the body in ridding itself of accumulated waste. I like to consider these two things -- an improved cardiovascular system and the cleansing effect of sweating -- the primary bene-fits of aerobic exercise. In addi-tion, there are a good many benefits which I like to call the secondary benefits of aerobic exercise because they occur largely as a result of the first two. Among these are a gradual lowering of the blood pressure; a gradual disappearance of cold feet and of leg cramps; frequently the end of constipation; weight loss where weight loss is desirable and weight gain where weight gain is in order; an end of insomnia; an enhanced sense of well-being, etc. Aerobic exercise ultimately makes the difference between health that is merely the absence of disease and health that is buoyantly vigorous. Once you have experienced the latter form of health, you will never again voluntarily settle for the former.

Apart from general health benefits, aerobic exercise is of special interest for the weight watcher and for those who want to give up sugar, caffeine and/or nicotine. It helps the weight watcher in several ways: 1. It burns up calories. 2. By reconditioning the heart and the network of veins and arteries, it improves blood circulation, and an improved blood circulation speeds up the break-down of fat deposits. 3. It reduces the appetite. By drawing much blood from the organs of the digestive system to the skeletal muscles which are involved in the exercise, it leaves the digestive tract in a sleepy, inactive condition, much as the rest of you feels drowsy and disinclined to action when the opposite happens; that is, when much blood is drawn away from the brain and the skeletal muscles to the digestive system after a big meal. But aerobic exercise helps to keep the weight watcher's appetite down in yet another way -- it gently raises the blood sugar level, and in so doing removes the sensations of hunger. It is a popular misconception that exercise increases the appetite. The opposite is true: though one may have been hungry before, one does not feel hungry for some time after exercise. This is of special significance for those who are afraid that they will put on weight if they quit smoking.

It is this raising of the blood sugar level that becomes the ex-smoker's and the reformed coffee drinker's or sugar addict's life-line to sanity when temptation assails him. If, when temptation gets to you, you resist it long enough to put on your running shoes and to break into your jogger's trot, you will have won another victory. It is quite unbelievable how quickly and how totally the craving for a smoke goes the moment you ease yourself into your favorite form of exercise.

Jogging, my choice of aerobic exercise, helped me in yet another way when I gave up smoking: every day, it seemed, my lungs breathed more freely, the wheezing grew fainter, and jogging became more of a joyful experience; and, after a relatively short time without smoking, my performance improved so much that I simply could not let myself down again by going back to my lung-clogging, fitness-destroying habit of smoking.

A word of caution. If you have not exercised regularly for some time, start slowly -- you cannot start too slowly – so as to give your body a chance to get itself ready. You'll pay dearly if you don't. I am not thinking of risks so drastic as a heart attack. The heart attack you may be spared even if you don't heed my advice. But there are lesser risks which you will not be spared -- all sorts of aches and pains, chiefly in those parts of the body that do most of the work -- legs and feet in jogging, rope skipping and bicycling; arms and back in rowing; arms and legs in tennis, etc. These aches and pains may become so crippling that you have to stop exercising for weeks or months, perhaps forever. Besides, if you push yourself too hard too fast, your exercise may turn into a painful chore instead of being the self-motivating fun it should and can be, and sooner or later you will be tempted to pack it in altogether; for no one, not even you, will stick to exercise forever that is not somehow fun.

Again I will pause. I have more to say about exercise -- how much of it you need, what kinds of exercise there are for you to choose from and more -- but I'll say it in a second appendix; for I don't want to slow you down too much while you find out about the major strategies.

Major strategy 5: Learn to relax through yoga and meditation. Every veteran smoker knows that, when his nerves are taut, he needs a smoke particularly badly -- just before a job interview, after a family quarrel, an undeserved dressing down at work, etc. Mr. Brean explains in some detail the connection between nerves and smoking in the chapter "Why You Really Smoke."

He concludes that, if one could get the tranquilizing effect of smoking without the adverse side effects, there would be little need for quitting. But, since it is not possible to separate the tranquilizer in the cigarette from the killer, you must quit. And you can take much of the sting out of quitting by reducing the need for the tranquilizing effect of smoking; that is, by ministering to your frayed nerves.

We have touched on various courses of action that can lead to calmer nerves. Stabilizing your sugar metabolism is one of them. Correcting deficiencies of nutrients that are essential for healthy nerves is another, especially the B-vitamins and certain minerals such as magnesium, potassium, and calcium. Aerobic exercise is another one. A vigorous game of tennis, a good run, a brisk half-hour walk or a long swim -- these are excellent tranquilizers that have no undesirable side effects. You are about to learn of yet another course of action that can improve the health of your nerves remarkably -- yoga and meditation.

A great many people still think of yoga and meditation as things for which there is no room in the daily routine of a sane citizen of the western world. They associate the two with the occult and with superstitious practices worthy of eastern gurus who spend much of their time standing on their heads or western drop-outs who barely qualify for membership in the society of ordinary human beings.

Much of the low esteem in which yoga and meditation are held in the western world can be attributed simply to lack of information; much of it, no doubt, is due to the contempt that is felt for some of the people who have championed the cause of yoga and meditation -- the flower children of yesterday or the drop- outs of today at one end of the scale; at the other end, those who have exploited the two practices, especially meditation, to enrich themselves. Fortunately the number of respectable in-betweeners is growing, those for whom yoga and meditation are neither means of escape nor source of enrichment, but rather a way of toning and relaxing both body and mind to make them healthier and better able to cope.

As for yoga, I used to think that to learn it, I would have to enrol in a formal yoga class. I was reluctant to do that because I was not sure that I could handle it or convinced that it would do me good. Nor did I like the idea of becoming a student again. The very thought of it put a damper on my desire to enrol, and I never did. But gradually, as I became better informed in other areas of health and healthful living, I pickedup bits of information about yoga incidentally, became more interested in it, and finally decided that I had at least to find out what it was and what it could do for me. So I bought some books on yoga and worked my way through them. When I had finished, most of the fog had cleared. Here is a brief summary of what I learned:

1. You can learn how to do yoga without formal instruction. With a good book, you can teach yourself yoga in your own living room.
2. Our schools condition us to think that doing things is worth while only if we do them with 100-per cent efficiency. Yoga made me realize how wrong this sort of attitude is. After all, though I do certain exercises only half as well as an sepert, I still benefit from doing them. Surely a little yoga is better than no yoga at all.
3. There is much more to yoga than standing on your head; in fact, standing on your head is only one of dozens of poses, and you may ignore it altogether if either it does not appeal to you or you cannot do it.
4. You may ignore any of the yoga poses that don't appeal to you. For your daily yoga routine, select those that do.
5. Certain breathing exercises are part of yoga. They are particularly good for the beginning non-smoker in the throes of withdrawal misery.

With yoga, as with so many things, "the proof of the pudding is in the eating." Try it for a few weeks and you will probably find yourself hooked on it as I did and continue to do. Among other things, yoga loosens stiff joints and relaxes tense nerves; it gently stimulates blood circulation; improved blood circulation, together with the breathing exercises, results in more efficient oxygen transportation to all parts of the body, including the brain, and a general defogging of the brain occurs; yoga relieves indigestion, constipation, insomnia, headaches and many other aches and pains; it gently massages vital organs and leaves them in better working order; a general improvement in body tone, in circulatory efficiency and in mental alertness gradually leads to more self-confidence and a more optimistic outlook on life. Of special interest to the smoker who wants to quit are the breathing exercises, which help to repair damaged lungs and to fight the temptation to light up, and calmer nerves, which result in a diminished dependence on the tranquilizing effect of smoking.

For the beginner who would like to give yoga a try in his own living room, I recommend Kareen Zebroff's ABC of Yoga. It contains 46 rather easy yoga poses and four breathing exercises. It offers clear and easy-to-follow instructions with each exercise and photographs to illustrate various stages of it. I used the book myself. Here is how I went about it. The first day I very quickly skimmed through the book trying all the 46 poses, one after another, to see whether I could do them. The second day I again started from the beginning, only this time I did no more than about 15 of the exercises. I spent a little more time on each, and I placed a check mark beside those that appealed to me. I did another 15 the following day, and the remaining 16 on the third day. Then I went through the whole book again, this time attending only to those exercises which I had honored with a check mark. From these I selected the 12 I liked best, and they became my standard yoga routine. I have since revised that routine several times, dropping some of the exercises and adding a few new ones with each revision. Now several decades later, I have a basic repertoire of 15. These I perform almost daily. If I happen to have little time, I go through the whole routine in as little time as eight minutes; if I am not rushed, I spend as much as twenty minutes to half an hour on it.

I have long since graduated to Kareen Zebroff's second book, "Advancing with Yoga and Nutrition." I handled it as I had handled the first one, and my present routine contains some exercises from both books. There are, by the way, a good many exercises in the second book which I can do only very badly or hardly at all. I waste no psychic energy worrying about them but stick to the ones which I can do reasonably well. And there are a great many of those. Every once in a while, when I feel really ambitious, I leaf through the two books again and I try myself at exercises which I either did not like or could not do earlier on. In the process my basic routine still undergoes an occasional revision.

Meditation has, as it were, come out. It is basically a technique of relaxing the mind and, through the mind, the body. Though many people who are deeply religious practice meditation -- in the Christian tradition, the equivalent of meditation is contemplation -- there is no direct connection between religion and meditation. It is a technique which the infidel can practice as well the believer. Further, meditation requires no special equipment: you need no incense to meditate, no crystal ball, no fetish. You don't need the stimulants of nicotine or caffeine to put you in the meditative state. On the contrary, meditation itself has freed many people from the addiction to these substances, and more and more are discovering that they can get"high" naturally on meditation itself.

But meditation is not just silly kid stuff. Very serious adults have practiced meditation in all ages, and many a cool-headed scientist or businessman has adopted it in our era as a technique that enables him to meet the stresses of modern life more efficiently. Meditation is for everyone -- for you and for me, for the young and for the old. You need no special talent to meditate, no exceptional intelligence.

Meditation does not make people lazy. Because some of the advocates of meditation have rejected the preoccupation with work and financial success so prevalent in the west, some people have concluded that meditation itself causes a disinclination to work. Quite the opposite is true: you will find that, if you meditate regularly, you will perform more efficiently whatever work you are engaged in. At the same time it would be wrong to think that meditation itself is a specific cure for either congenital or acquired laziness.

When I mention meditation, people often ask me, "Just what do you meditate about?" This question, it seems, is prompted by the fact that the term "meditation" denotes both "to think intensely about something" and "to practice a technique of physical and mental relaxation," and the questioner assumes that the two must be interchangeable. The two meanings, however, are not connected in any other way than that they happen to lodge in the same word; in fact, "to meditate" in our sense is, as much as possible, not to think about anything at all.

Meditation, finally, is no more the monopoly of any one school of meditation than social wisdom is the monopoly of any one political party. Don't let the partisans of TM convince you that theirs is the only true form of meditation. Nothing against TM. The technique is good and TM teachers usually teach it well; but you do not need to invest $ 300 in a TM course in order to learn how to meditate. Allan Watt's Meditation, an inexpensive paperback, will get you there. So will How to Meditate, another paperback, or the directions I am about to give you in the following four basic steps of meditation:

1. Pick a time and a place where you will not be disturbed for half an hour; a reasonably quiet place, if

possible.

2. Sit on a couch or in an easy-chair. Wriggle yourself into a comfortable position. Place your hands loosely beside your thighs or in your lap. Instead of sitting up, you may lie on your back. But do not lie either on an uncarpeted floor or on your bed: the former is not comfortable enough to relax; the latter is likely to be too comfortable, and you may fall asleep before you get around to meditate. If you want to lie on your back, lie on a rug.

3. Once you are physically comfortable, get yourself mentally comfortable. How? By being as passive as you can. From here on, stop "trying"; just let things happen. You do not even have to believe in meditation: as long as you do not sit there worrying whether it will work, it will.

4. Step 4 differs from school to school. I'll give you several variations of it. Try them all; then pick the one which works best for you. But do not mix them. Decide which one you are going to use before you get ready to meditate and then stick to it.

Variation 1: Close your eyes. Slowly take a deep breath and as slowly exhale. Now shift your attention from whatever is in or on your mind to your breathing. Feel your breath enter your lungs and feel your chest expand with it; then feel your chest contract as your breath exits. For a little while, do no more than attend to your breathing. If your thoughts put up a fight, if they refuse to yield the center stage of your awareness, which has been undisputedly theirs for as long as they can remember, simply ignore them and go on paying attention to your breathing. In no time at all there will be peace upstairs.

After you have observed yourself breathe for the duration of a dozen breaths or more, start attaching a pair of syllables to each breath -- the syllable ONE as it enters your lungs and the syllable TWO as it leaves. You may either "think" or "gently mumble" these syllables. The main purpose of the procedure is to help you break away from your normal pattern of conscious thought.

One of two things may happen -- either you lose yourself completely in a state of mind which is not conscious of itself or anything else, or you become conscious of certain thoughts -- the fact that you are punctuating each breath with the syllables ONE-TWO, the fact that you have stopped paying attention to your breath, the fact that you are meditating, etc. The state of mind which is not conscious of itself or anything else is the state you want to be in. Paradoxically, the minute you know that you are in it, you are no longer in it; for then you have become conscious again. However, when you *do* become conscious, all you need to do is return to your point of departure; that is, mumble or think ONE-TWO, ONE-TWO, etc., again as you feel your breath enter and leave your lungs. In no time at all, you will lose yourself again. Occasionally a third thing may happen -- you may drift off to sleep. No cause for concern unless you oversleep the end of your lunch break and don't get back to work on time. Till you can be fairly sure that you won'r fall asleep and oversleep your next commitment, it may be a good idea to set a timer. Otherwise, do not get upset when you become aware that you have fallen asleep, calmly take note of it and return to your point of departure.

Keep this up for about 20 minutes. Then slowly move your arms, your legs, your whole body, stretch, and open your eyes. Sit for a few more seconds. Then get up slowly, ready to step back into the cycle of your daily routine. You will feel wonderfully refreshed and rested.

Variation 2: Instead of paying attention to your reathing, "focus" your attention on a pleasant sense object -- a flower,the flame of a lit candle, a pretty picture. Do not think about about the object or anything else but confidently allow things to go their way. Breathe normally through your nose. If conscious or semi-conscious thoughts continue to call for your attention, refuse to oblige them. Keep looking at your object. If, or when, your eyes feel the least bit fatigued, gently permit them to close. With eyesclosed, try so gently that it is like not trying at all to visualize the object you were looking at before you allowed your eyes to close. That's all. When you become "conscious," return to your point of departure. Continue for what feels like 20 minutes. Come out of it as in Variation 1 above.

Variation 3: This time the aid for breaking away from conscious thought is a sound -- a mantra. Partisans of TM will warn you that no mantra will work for you except the one a trained TM teacher assigns to you in a personal interview. The mantra so assigned will work, no doubt about it; but so will any sound you find pleasant and soothing. It may be a single syllable, a word, a phrase, or a whole sentence. It may be sound without meaning or sound with meaning. Try the sound Allan Watts uses – I use it myself -- ahm... ahmmm... ahmmmm Chant it softly at various pitches, till you find a pitch that "turns you on." Softly intone the sound at that pitch for a minute or two and then let it fade, but continue to hold an image of it in your mind as you did with candle flame or flower. If you become conscious of having lost the sound, return to your point of departure.

Variation 4: This is the way of "getting there" which I use when I feel tense. It consists of two phases -- one that relaxes the body and one that relaxes the mind. The body part is much like Karen Zebroff's "sponge." (ABC of Yoga, p. 100). I lie on my back, legs slightly apart. To begin with, I shake my body loose and wriggle myself into a comfortable position. Then I think myself through a routine of relaxing my body part by part. I start with my toes. I tense the muscles in my toes gently so as to become fully aware of them. After a couple of seconds I relax them and "forget" about them as though they were no longer there. Next I "concentrate" on my feet. I gently turn them left and right, till I have the full feel of them; then I let go and "forget" about them. This way I slowly work my way up my whole body -- my legs, my thighs, my behind, etc. By the time I get to my scalp, my whole body is so completely relaxed that I am hardly aware of its existence. To conclude this phase, I mentally sweep over my whole body once more, this time without moving a muscle, without tensing a tendon. I start at my toes and in one slow but continuous sweep I pass over my body thinking to myself, "... my thighs ... my knees ... my chest ... my shoulders ... so relaxed I can't feel they are there."

Here is how I go about relaxing my mind. I first wipe away all conscious thought. If I miss a few fragments of thought with the first sweep of the mental eraser, I don't trouble to sweep again; they will soon disappear by themselves. Next I fetch from my memory files a place or scene that is ringed with pleasant emories -- the hammock in my grandparents' backyard, a hide-out among the rocks by the sea, a boat out in the bay at sunset -- and I project that place or scene on my inner screen. I savor the pleasant memories that surround it. Otherwise I treat it much as I treated the candle flame or the flower after I closed my eyes. It becomes my point of departure. About 20 minutes later I return to reality as in Variation 1 above.

A few points to remember. These directions will get you there. If you want more detailed instructions, read the excellent chapter "The `How' of Meditation" in How to Meditate. The one thing you must not do when you set out to meditate is try to meditate. The only thing you may consciously do is to direct your attention to your breathing, the flower, the flame or the mantra and then "get out of the way." Whatever happens is good, as long as you do not try to make things happen. When y ou become conscious of any mental activity -- whether it is a thought your mind has been chasing or even the fact that you are meditating, gently detach yourself and return to your point of departure. And -- meditate regularly.

Meditation is credited with many positive effects on the meditator's physiology, his brain-wave activity, his ability to concentrate, etc. Of particular interest for the smoker getting ready to quit is the fact that meditation, if practiced regularly, calms nerves; and calmer nerves means a lessening of the need for the tranquilizing effect of smoking. Why not give it a try? Meditation is the most effortless one of all the major strategies. It is cheap. All it costs is a little of your time. Besides, it is a very effective tranquilizer without any harmful side effects. So -- no risks, but much to gain.

Major strategy 6: Practice the technique of auto-suggestion. Whatever the label -- autosuggestion, auto-genic training, self-hypnosis -- all these terms really name the same thing -- a technique intended to enlist the support of the unconscious for a conscious purpose. If practiced conscien- tiously, it can produce fantastic results.

The scientific community of the day was shocked when Freud first dared to tell the world that man was not really master in his own house; that reason was but the puppet dancing on strings manipulated by a cunning and capricious puppet master, the Unconscious. In due time, however, the learned relented and
Freud's doctrine became the dominant new creed.

It is still much with us -- the notion that man's best

laid plans gang oft astray and his most cherished hopes are thwarted owing to the machinations of the unconscious part of his mental make-up. And the general assumption is that the unconscious is enemy rather than friend. But we are approaching the end of the tunnel. We have begun to understand that the unconscious is not our enemy, whatever its power over our feelings, our attitudes and what we like to think of as rational thought; and that, though we be the puppets, we are not nearly as helpless as we have permitted ourselves to believe. In the following pages, in fact, you will be shown how you, the puppet, can learn to manipulate the puppet master so as to make of him your most powerful ally for your impending fight against smoking.

Think of the unconscious as something like a computer that stores every bit of information regarding all experiences you ever undergo. Every bit of stored information is instantly available. Now, imagine that a fragment of a tune drifts in on you from somewhere. Your conscious does not remember either the tune or the setting in which you encountered it. But your internal computer instantly matches the signal with the appropriate memory file and instantly you experience feelings similar to the ones you experienced when you first encountered the tune. Or you pick up a sensation of smell. You cannot place it, but your internal computer matches it with the right bit of memory and instantly you feel nostalgic or happy or frightened without knowing why. Or, for no apparent reason, you feel drawn to a stranger you meet for the first time. If you could follow the flurry of activity in your internal computer, you might learn that it matched certain gestures of the stranger with gestures that were typical of your grandfather. Since the signal from the past came wrapped in associations of warmth and security, presto you felt warm and secure before this stranger. It seems the unconscious gets into the act long before the conscious has a chance to respond.

One of the most exciting things to have come out of recent psychological and parapsychological research is the realization that we can alter the programming that has gone into our unconscious. We may not be able actually to erase an old signal; but, by programming in a new signal that is contrary to the old one in intent, we can take the wind out of the old one's sails; and, if the new signal is strong enough, we can actually have contrary action initiated. To illustrate, for reasons which my conscious does not understand, I panic when a horse comes near me. Relatives, owners of a large farm, have several riding horses. I like the sight of them from a safe distance, but I dare not go near them, let alone ride one of them. This disqualifies me from the frequent horseback excursions which all the participants seem to enjoy immensely. I envy them, but my fear of horses prevents me from joining them. Then someone shows me how to program into my internal computer a signal contrary to and stronger than that fear. The unbelievable happens: I become part of the horseback team. The ecstasy of it!

How then do I go about programming new information into my internal computer? For, one thing is certain -- it won't take any direct orders from me. I know, for instance, that there is no reason why I should panic at the thought of a speech I have to deliver: I am thoroughly familiar with the subject matter and I have prepared the speech well. Yet I am all nerves. It is obvious that my unconscious is playing tricks on me again. But, no matter how many times I tell myself that there is nothing to worry about, I continue to tremble.

To get through to the internal computer, I must wait till the unconscious relaxes its tight security. It does that when the conscious mind goes to sleep; but then I am asleep too and I cannot attempt any re-programming. Fortunately there are other moments when the nconscious relaxes its watchfulness enough to become susceptible to suggestion while I myself am still conscious enough to take advantage of the situation   I have in mind those magic moments that occur between waking and sleeping, morning and evening: the dividing line between reality and dream begins to blur but I am still conscious enough to transmit a message, which I thought out and formulated earlier, while fully awake.

Specifically, this is how to go about it. You have gone to bed and the lights are out. You have closed your eyes. Now lie on your back and wriggle yourself into the most comfortable position you can find. Relax. If you wish, you may go through the physical relaxation routine described in "variation 4" above. Otherwise, just take a deep breath slowly, and as slowly exhale. Then start talking to your unconscious. Think of it as your unconscious partner and address it thus:

"Partner, I want to stop smoking, but I cannot do it alone. I need your help. If I quit, we shall both benefit. So let's work on it together and, when the time comes, benefit from it together."

Conclude the session by visualizing yourself vividly as a non-smoker, taking deep breaths of clean air into lungs no longer raspy with smoke damage; visualize your spouse smiling happily because your breath and your clothes no longer reek of smoke; visualize yourself running effortlessly up several flights of stairs, your breath coming and going smoothly; visualize yourself as a non-smoker in any situation that appeals to you. Fall asleep with the picture on your inner screen. Do the same thing in the morning when you wake.

The whole procedure need not take more than three or four minutes. Do it faithfully evening and morning for perhaps a month and then "get out of the way" confident that your unconscious partner got the message and is going to act upon it. Don't worry if sometimes you fall asleep before you finish your little act or if, in the morning, you forget all about it not to remember till you are up and away. An occasional lapse like this will not defeat your intent.

You don't even have to believe in auto-suggestion. It helps if you believe in it; for, one tends to do better what one believes in. But it will work even if you don't believe in it. And when you finally get through to your unconscious partner and (s)he gets into the act, you will know: you will of sudden feel as though someone or something had infused you with new courage. Instead of the old fear of failure, there will be the sudden certainty that this time you will do it.

This strategy of auto-suggestion by itself could conceivably do the trick of getting you to quit. It has done so for other people. But there is no way of knowing in advance whether it will be all it takes for you to get ready. And, since this is going to be your last try, you do not want any half-measures. Practice all the strategies -- those designed to rebuild your fitness and health to the point where your body won't need smoking any more and the strategy of auto-suggestion: the latter will get you launched on the road to quitting; the former will make it easy for you to stay on that road, much easier than you found it at any other time in the past.

V

MINOR STRATEGIES

The major strategies discussed in the previous chapters take time: one does not eat oneself back into good health in a few days, no matter how good the diet; and the results of years without exercise are not undone by a week of jogging or swimming, however vigorous. So don't be impatient, and do not let the length of the preparation period discourage you. Having tried the instant approach without success before, you must make up your mind to do things differently this time if you hope to get there.

Don't let the prospect of having to go on smoking for another month or two discourage you either. You have smoked for years; another couple of months hopefully won't mean the end of you. What matters is that you do get yourself unhooked at last. And you will, if you do things right. Besides, you may take comfort from the fact that, with every bit of improvement in your fitness and your health, your body will be better able to compensate for the harm smoking does to you. I know a veteran smoker who every now and then decides to quit. The moment he quits, he starts to jog; and the moment he stops quitting, he stops jogging. "What's the good of jogging," he argues, "if I smoke again?" I can't get him to understand that his need for exercise is greater, not less, when he smokes; for, exercise will undo at least part of the damage he inflicts on his system by smoking.

At the same time there are a few things you may do to minimize the damage of smoking. Write to the Center for Disease Control, National Clearing House for Smoking and Health, Attention Tar and Nicotine, Atlanta, Georgia, 30333, for a US government pamphlet that tells you how to minimize the effects of tar and nicotine. In the meantime, treat yourself to some extra vitamins -- C and B1 to compensate for losses of them due to smoking; A, because it is necessary for the health of the mucous membrane that lines the nasal cavity, the mouth and the rest of the respiratory tract. Consider rolling your own cigarettes. If you do, you won't light up quite so often because it takes more effort to roll a cigarette than to reach for a ready-made one. Moreover, you will inhale fewer chemicals. At the very least you will avoid the chemicals put into regular cigarettes to keep them burning when you put them down. Finally, you can reduce the damage of smoking by reducing smoking itself. I am not suggesting that you should slowly wean yourself from say 50 cigarettes a day to none at all. For most people this slow-torture approach does not work. It did not work for me. What I have in mind is a gradual reduction from two or three packs a dayto only a pack, on the assumption that a daily 20 does you less harm than a daily 50; and that, when the time comes to quit completely, it will be less of a shock to graduate to zero from 20 than from 50.

Reducing your daily cigarette consumption moderately does not take a super-effort of willpower. For one thing, if you adopt the major strategies discussed in the previous chapter, your cigarette consumption will automatically go down; for, as your health improves, your dependence on cigarettes will lessen and you will light up less often. More specifically, you will need your nicotine "fix" much less desperately if you stabilize your blood sugar and if you exercise. And you can make the labor of reducing your nicotine intake easier by playing a few games with yourself.

Here are some of the games that helped me cut down. Play them if you think they will help you; if not, devise some games of your own. The most effective one I found was to put distance between my cigarettes and me. The trick is to find the right distance: if it is too short, you will traverse it too easily; if too long, it may lead to anger and frustration and ultimately \provoke you to smoke more instead of less. For me the right distance turned out to be the distance between my second-floor \ apartment and my car. Again and again, the following mini-drama would enact itself: Without instructions from my conscious self, my right hand would reach for the pack of cigarettes that was not there. Then the conscious recollection would burst in on me, "O, they are in the car!" My first reaction would be one of annoyance. "Nuisance," I'd grumble to myself; "guess I'll have to go down to get one of those blasted things." And sometimes I'd do just that. At other times, however, the internal monologue might continue this way: "But, can't I go on reading (or writing or watching t.v. or whatever I happened to be doing) without a cigarette for a few more minutes? It is not as though I can't have a cigarette. All I have to do is dash downstairs and get one. But I feel too lazy just now to run down. Maybe I'll try to go on reading for a while...." Quite often I would argue myself into settling back to whatever I was doing and actually "forget" about smoking for minutes, for tens of minutes.

Another game I played was roll my own cigarettes. Sometimes the bother of having to roll one would be enough to keep me from smoking for a little while. Or I would deliberately seek out places where I could not smoke, such as the library, a church or the home of a friend who is allergic to cigarette smoke. And I got myself a little toy savings bank, into which I would slip a dime every time I'd manage to stay off smoking for a quarter of an hour or more. The accumulated dimes I could use recklessly to buy something I wanted but which my sense of thrift would not let me buy. These games helped. The last few weeks before I quit I was down to less than a pack a day from between two and three packs a day.

One more minor strategy before I conclude this section. Take pen and paper, even now, and jot down all the reasons you can think of for wanting to give up smoking. Be brief. No need to write sentences or aragraphs. A word or a short phrase will do in each instance. Then put the list somewhere where you can be sure you will find it again when you need it. Every time you can think of yet another reason why you should quit, go and add that reason to your list. A few minutes from now; tonight, as you'll be thinking about giving up smoking; tomorrow; next week -- you'll be surprised how many more reasons for quitting you will come up with. It's like compiling a list of things to take on a trip. The only sure way not to forget anything is to start the list days or weeks ahead of time and to add to it every time you think of something else to take. I used to keep two copies of my list -- a rough copy, on a file card in my wallet, and a finished copy in my desk. Whenever I thought of another reason, I'd jot it down on the rough copy and later I'd transfer the new entry to the finished copy. The final count was 31 reasons for quitting.

I still have that list, and every once in a while I look at it and I feel good. While I was getting ready to quit, I read that list once or twice every day. I'd read it slowly, lingering a little on each reason and "day-dream-inh " of the day when that reason would not apply any longer. Thus I added to the impact of the auto-suggestion program, making sure that my unconscious partner understood not merely that I wanted to quit but also that there were a good many good reasons why I should.

VI

YOU ACTUALLY QUIT

You have been preparing yourself by practicing the major strategies for some time. You have been sending appeals to your unconscious partner for some time. Now it is only a question of a little more time before you will feel ready to take the last step. Quite suddenly, some day soon, you will feef ready.

If you don't believe me, let me remind you that you have experienced in other areas of life the sudden kind of readiness which I have in mind. Some chore you ought to do but which, for reasons you cannot fathom, you have not been able to get yourself to do. It may be a borrowed book to be returned to its owner. Every time you see that book, you feel guilty. Every time you see it you mumble to yourself that the next time you go to the part of town where the owner of the book lives you must remember to take it with you. But you forget. And you forget again. Then, one day, you realize that you have once again gone to "that part of town" without remembering to take the book with you. And all of a s udden there is no more putting it off. In a burst of angry readiness you grab it, hop into your car and take it to the owner's hous   Your daily mumbling "I've got to take that book back" finally Got hrough to your unconscious partner. When (s)he gets in The act, things get done.

For you, it may not be a book to be returned. It may be taking the car to a garage to have a broken mirror replaced or repotting a plant that has grown too big for its pot or starting to organize the notes you have been col-lecting for your thesis. As often as thought of the chore flashes across the horizon of your consciousness, you have some excuse for putting it off. It's not that you don't have time. We somehow always find time for things we really want to do. You just cannot "work up enough steam" to get at it. But daily you think about it, feel guilty about it, mumble to yourself that you just have to get it done. Then, one day, you suddenly experience that burst of readiness which indicates that you have finally got through to your unconscious partner. The cobwebs of motivational confusion have disappeared. You get the job done without further delay.It seems there's "nothing to it," and you cannot understand any More how you could have procrastinated so long.

So it will be with the job of quitting. Some day, quite suddenly, you will feel ready. The fog of emotional conflict will have cleared -- doubts gone, self-pity gone, and gone the panic at the thought of never having another cigarette. Instead there will be the calm certainty that you can and will do it.

Your unconscious partner has ways of letting you know when you are ready. A friend of mine, a heavy smoker who had been "thinking" about giving up moking for some time, ran out of cigarettes at a bridge party. He started to "borrow" cigarettes from his wife. When her supply was beginning to run low, she snapped at him that she was sick of him bumming cigarettes from her and never paying her back. He snapped back. Tempers heated. In a burst of anger he threw the cigarette he had been about to light at her hissing, "...last time I'll bum a cigarette from you. I am gonna quit." That was several weeks ago, and he has not had a smoke since. Of course the quarrel with his wife was not what made him quit; it was merely the occasion for readiness to announce itself.

Here is how readiness made itself known to me. I mentioned earlier that during my last few weeks of smoking I had managed to cut down to less than a pack a day. I felt good about that. Then something happened to send my cigarette consumption soaring again. On my way home from work, I had rushed into a store to buy a carton of cigarettes. When I ripped it open at home, I realized that I had made a double blunder: I had bought "regular" instead of "king-size" and I had bought the wrong brand. If someone else had done this to me, I could have been ready to kill. In a fit of white-hot fury, I lit one of the cursed little things and -- yes, you guessed it -- I could not get a smoke out of it. I smoked one cigarette after another till, in less than three hours, I had finished all but three cigarettes of one pack. Then something clicked. I knew I had come to a parting of the ways: it was either back to more han two packs a day or quit. At that instant I knew that slipping back was much more terrifying than quitting altogether. I threw away the three cigarettes that remained in the pack and I put the other nine packs away in a drawer -- out of reach, out of sight, out of mind. At that moment, just over forty years ago, I became a non-smoker.

It would be wrong to assume that the double blunder of buying the wrong size and the wrong brand of cigarettes made me so furious that I quit at last. The frustration of the wrong cigarettes merely became the occasion for readiness to make itself known. I have often wondered whether the whole thing was not perhaps engineered deliberately by my unconscious partner so as to bring home to me the fact that I was ready.

Your unconscious partner may not send you so specific a "sign" to let you know when you are ready to quit; it may just send you a general feeling of readiness and leave it to you to select the day when you will become a non-smoker. Don't be in too much of a hurry to get going. Give the major strategies time to "take." I suggest that you allow at least two months, possibly even three. Besides, do not quit a few days before exams, the night before a big party to be given or attended, where many people will be smoking, before any period of major stress. A quiet weekend, no smoking relatives coming to visit, no due-on-Monday job of an essay or a report to get up-tight over, no crisis of any kind anticipated -- that's the time to quit. Make Friday noon your zero hour. Somehow you will last through the afternoon. Come 4:30, you can go home to the security of two days of splendid isolation, during which you can get yourself well launched on the road to quitting. If your own home is not the ideal place to spend those first two or three days in, consider going away for the weekend. You might spend the weekend with friends or relatives who would be in favor of your project, or you may simply sign yourself into a motel armed with several books that you have long wanted to read. Consider cashing in a day or two of vacation time saved up at work so as to extend your weekend to include Monday and Tuesday. The weekend you quit smoking is one of the most important weekends in your life. Make it as pleasant and relaxed a weekend as possible.

Weekend or midweek, workday or holiday, whether your unconscious partner chooses the moment for your last cigarette or you do so yourself, when you finally jump off the treadmill of addiction and start walking the road to freedom, you will feel from the beginning that this time it is going to be different. No doubt the first few days are going to be difficult again, but you are well prepared. Mr. Brean's How to Stop Smoking contains an excellent day-by-day preview of the first two weeks of the journey. (Chapter 10, pp. 115 ff.) Take it with you and read it as you go along. In How We Quit Smoking, Health and Welfare Canada's collection of 78 case histories, you will find many tricks and tactics that might prove useful to you. And continue to practice the major strategies for a while. Practicing them should not be difficult any more; they should be second nature to you now. Every night and every morning transmit to your unconscious partner a vivid visualization of yourself as a well-established non-smoker; give a wide berth to substances that could unbalance your sugar metabolism; continue to eat wholesome food, to exercise, and to practice your technique of relaxation. These strategies prepared you for the ordeal of quitting and they will see you through it.

There follow a few more tips for the fledgling non-smoker. To begin with, let it be understood that not all the tricks which others have found useful will work for you. Mr.Brean, for instance, suggests that you should let friend and foe know that you are about to quit smoking; for, as he puts it,

"The thought of all the derisive laughter you will get for giving in may well carry you over the crisis, which is the reason why you should let others know about what you are doing." (How To Stop Smoking, p. 82)

This may work for some people, but surely it won't work for everybody. For you it may, in fact, be counter-productive in that it may add another stress to an already stressful situation -- the fear of losing face before your friends and of being taunted by your enemies if you should break down. A friend of mine, about to get himself launched on one of many attempts to quit, bragged it up before relatives, friends and acquaintances and entered bets with some of them on his becoming and remaining a non-smoker. The fear of losing the bets, he hoped, would provide the extra incentive he needed to quit and to stay quit. He lost both his bets and his battle against nicotine. As for you, you will have to decide for yourself whether it is better for you to suffer in silence or to let all the world know. Weight Watchers of America think the first of the alter-natives the better one. So do I. Mr. Brean, on the other hand, believes in the second one.

Here is another question which you will have to answer for yourself -- whether you should carry cigarettes

with you after you quit. Some people do so to keep panic
at bay; I did not, for I was not certain that, if a cigarette
were within reach, I might not weaken. I had done so
before, and I was notgoing to take any chances.

You yourself will have to decide, too, whether you
should take it a day at a time or set your sights for orever.
I recommend the forever method. During my earlier
attempts I had used the one-day-at-a-time approach.
Once I had actually kept a log, in which I entered time
gone without smoking; at first in hours, later in days, and
finally in weeks. For a while the log seemed to help. It
became both incentive and reward. Sometimes I could
not wait to get back to it to make my entries of s o many
smokeless hours or days. During my last and final
attempt to quit, I set my sights for forever from the start;
in fact,"forever" was part of the message I transmitted to
my unconscious partner. And that, I am sure, made the
difference between merely giving up smoking and giving
up both smoking and wanting to smoke. It was as though
the secret agents of temptation, having clearly understood
that this time I wanted to quit for good, realized that they
had no chance and threw in the towel.

As for using food to pamper and to reward yourself
with while in the throes of quitting -- anything goes provided it does not lessen your chances of remaining a non-
smoker. Spoil yourself then, but do so wisely. Go for the
filet mignon or the chateaubriand with vegetables, baked
potato and sour cream rather than candy, ice-cream, chocolate, coffee or sugar-rich soft drinks. Food of the filet
mignon type may, at the worst, translate itself into a few
unwanted pounds; but that is something you need not
worry about till later since it does not prejudice your
chances of remaining a non-smoker. First things first:
quit now, and if you should put on a few pounds, get to
work on them later, when you are safely established as a
non-smoker. Food -- I am not sure it deserves to be

called food -- such as candy, ice-cream, chocolate, etc., is a different matter. It can seriously upset your sugar metabolism, and in doing so make it difficult for you, if not impossible, to stay off cigarettes. Remember what I told you about blood sugar and smoking in Chapter II, in particular about blood sugar and willpower. Hands off candy, therefore, and chocolate, ice-cream and soft drinks -- any food, in fact, that contains white sugar and white flour.

You probably know from past experience that the first few days are, though very bad in some ways, not really the most critical ones. True, you think of cigarettes almost constantly. You experience all sorts of withdrawal symptoms -- you feel dizzy, you break out in cold sweats, your head aches, your hands tremble, etc. And you go through a variety of mental withdrawal symptoms -- you are nervous, irritable and generally hard to live with, for yourself and for others; you cannot concentrate; you can't remember things. Yet, in spite of all your misery, you experience a sense of achievement that keeps your morale high.

For most people, the most critical time comes after the first three or four days; a time, ironically, when the very worst of the withdrawal misery begins to subside. Temptation gradually shifts from the more tangible forms of physical craving to subtler forms that are more difficult to combat. Let's examine some of them so that you will be the better prepared to deal with them when they assail you.

Sometimes temptation comes in the guise of a simple lapse of memory. Of a sudden, you cannot remember one good reason why you should go on with this nonsense of quitting. That's when your list will come in handy. Pull it out and read it slowly, reason after cogent reason, till you remember.

At times temptation comes as what I call withdrawal depression, something that can so befuddle you that you begin to doubt altogether whether you ever seriously wanted to quit. Everything about quitting suddenly seems unreal, even your list, and you cannot work up enough steam to pull out that list and to read it. It is not unlike a lapse into real depression. The victim of it -- only yesterday he was cheerful and optimistic; today, though nothing has changed in his personal circumstances -- his wife still loves him, his debts are no worse than they were yesterday and his job is still secure -- today, as I was about to say, wherever he looks, there seems to be gloom, the whole universe appears to be hostile and there seems to be nothing worth living for. One thing that can help the victim of depression to ride it out is consciously to remind himself that the apparent change in his circumstances is really only a change of his perception of them -- probably something gone wrong temporarily in his brain chemistry that has thrown things out of focus. The best proof that the causes of most depressions are internal, not external, is the fact that depression often strikes when all is well, rather than at times of crisis. Though the reminder that, however hopeless things may seem, sooner or later the universe will be right side up again. may not cure the depression, it helps the victim to ride it out. Similarly the ex-smoker caught in a bout of withdrawal depression should consciously remind himself that, in spite of what he is experiencing -- some sort of temporary irrationality due to a disturbance in his brain chemistry -- he does want to give up smoking; if he hangs on only for a little while, the fog will clear and he will know again in every fiber of his being how desperately he wants to quit. How he would hate and despise himself if he awoke from the momentary delusion. a cigarette stuck between his lips! It helps further to remind himself that the withdrawal depression inevitably burns itself out, usually in a matter of minutes. Then his misery will be over and he will feel proud again to be a non-smoker.

One of the most subtle agents in the secret service of temptation is self-pity. She comes whispering that you are the lonely martyr, abandoned by all, and now deprived even of your last comfort -- a cigarette. To arm yourself against this one of temptation's agents, remember that the thoughts you admit to your consciousness about a certain issue determine to a large extent how you feel about that issue. If you permit yourself to think that quitting is the ultimate sacrifice, you will end up feeling the martyr; if, instead, you nudge yourself gently into thinking that quitting is really the beginning of a new you, something that you have wanted for years, you will experience moments of ecstasy instead of feeling sorry for yourself.

Doubt is another one of temptation's agents. Her main argument is that it cannot be done. "Once hooked on cigarettes," she whispers, "always hooked. Millions of smokers have tried to quit only to discover, after weeks of needless misery, that they could not do it. What makes you think you are so different?" If you let her get as much as a toe in the doorway to your consciousness, you are in for trouble. Therefore counterattack at once. Shut the door in her face. Remind yourself that, if there are millions who have tried to quit and failed, there are also millions who have succeeded. You are going to be one of them. Close your eyes for a few minutes and day-dream of yourself as a permanently established non-smoker.

Yet another one of temptation's agents is Mr. False Courage. He is a super-salesman. His sales pitch is that, having shown to yourself and to all the world how surcharged you are with willpower, you may now permit yourself the luxury of an occasional puff. "Go on," he drawls, "have a puff; superman that you are, one puff cannot throw you." Don't fall for it. If you do, you will have another puff some time and another. And, just to prove to yourself how strong you really are, you will have a whole cigarette. The fact that you don't imme-diately revert to smoking 50 a day or more reassures you that all is still well. Meanwhile Mr. False Courage sits in the sidelines waiting. He knows that time is on his side. "Never fails," you hear him whisper to his colleagues, "get them to have that one puff, and the rest will take care of itself." Fear grips you that he might be right. But you have another cigarette -- just this one more; then you will quit again. "After all," you rationalize, "even if I have another cigarette or two before I quit again, what's a couple of cigarettes compared to the hundreds I used to smoke?"

The point, of course, is not how few cigarettes you smoke now; the point is that you have let temptation break through your defenses, a fact which has given it a new lease on life while it has seriously weakened your self-confidence. It won't be long before you will drop the pretense of rationalizing altogether. For a few more days you may keep your cigarette consumption down and feel that, though you did not manage to quit \altogether, you have gained much by cutting down to only a few ciga-rettes a day. But it is only a question of time. The next moment of crisis will see you back where you left off -- at 50 or 60 a day. And now and then you will day-dream again of a time when you will really quit.

Remember, whichever one of her many disguises tempta-tion approaches you in, the best way to fight her is not to let her engage you in a conversation in the first place. Treat temptation as you treat (or should treat) TV. A program which you really wanted to watch has just ended. Another is coming on. Walking away is easy if you do it before the new show has had a chance to get to you. In like manner, temptation will have no power over you if you flick the switch and walk away the minute it flashes up on your inner screen.

But now for a few down-to-earth, practical hints, which will help you either to avoid or to weather some of the crises, major and minor, that lie ahead.

1. Carry something to chew -- sugarless gum, a tooth-pick, a handful of nuts, etc. When in company, have something for your hands to play with -- a pen, a book, a piece of jewelry, a set of keys, a small notebook. It will be only for a little while. You were not born with the need to "handle" a cigarette. This need is an acquired need, a learned pattern of behavior, and anything that can be learned can also be unlearned.

2. When things get bad, put on your running shoes and jog a mile; if you cannot do that, go for a brisk walk.

3. Keep busy. Keeping busy at work you will will endear yourself to your boss and to your supervisor. At home, take time out for your favorite hobby. Even when I was a smoker, not trying to quit, I could get so absorbed in making things of wood, my favorite hobby, that I could totally forget about smoking for an hour or more; and sometimes, though I wanted a cigarette, I could not be bothered to light one because I was too impatient to get on with what I was doing.

4. Do some deep-breathing exercises. Go open a window And take half a dozen deep breaths of fresh air.

5. Go to bed. Early evening can be a bad time, especially after supper, the time when you read the paper. If the urge to smoke threatens to overwhelm you, take the easy way out - fully legitimate in this case -- and slip off to bed. The fact that, for most smokers, bed is not associated with smoking helps. If you can fall asleep, you've got it made; for there is nothing like sleep to defuse temptation. If you can't, just lie on your back, take a few deep breaths and meditate.

6. Read a book which you can't put down. Combine reading With being in bed. When you begin to feel drowsy, simply put the book down and "let go."

7. Avoid excitement that can be avoided. Card games are occasions when people smoke more than their usual quota. Worked up by the game, they need a smoke to calm down. But the game continues, and one cigarette is hardly put ou When taut nerves demand another.. Much the same is true of watching hockey, baseball or football, live or on t.v. Whether your side wins or loses, you are likely to get all worked up and to want cigarette after cigarette to calm down. For a little while at least, fill an evening with reading a book instead of playing bridge or watching a game;or go to see a good movie at a theater where you are not permitted to smoke; or go to a concert; or visit friends who do not smoke.

You should also refuse to be drawn into an argument. Keep your mouth shut and, if at all possible,walk away; for, if you stay, you are as likely as not to put in your two bits' worth in spite of the best intentions. One word leads to another, adrenalin begins to flow and tempers heat. Most ordinary quarrels have no rational basis. They feed on themselves. When they are over, and when tempers have cooled, the participants feel embarrassed at having allowed themselves to slip into senseless fury. No, let them taunt -- husband or wife, father or mother, son or daughter -- you cannot lose a battle which you do not join. And, though you were to enter the fray and win, would you want to bargain away your chances of winning your war against smoking for the prospect of a victory in a petty argument? How bitter that victory would taste if, when you should come to your senses, you'd find a cigarette stuck between your fingers.

8. Avoid any other situation that might trigger the smoking urge. For a while at least, stay away from the crowd that gathers in a smoke-filled lunch room. Go for

a brisk walk instead. Take deep lungfuls of fresh air. Instead of feeling sorry for yourself, feel sorry for the poor benighted smokers. Not long ago you were one of them. How you wished then to be a non-smoker. Now you are. Yes, you've done it. Keep walking, man; keep walking, woman. Perhaps you should avoid the company of smokers altogether, at least for the first few days. You may not be able to avoid them altogether at work, but you can stay away from the bridge table or from the party at a friend's house, where most people smoke. A good many smokers, though they profess to be your friends, do not really want you to quit as long as they themselves remain hooked. You know from experience how people, who have never before thought of offering you a cigarette, suddenly become generosity itself when they find out that you are trying to quit. You are much better off without their generosity, and you do not need their cheerless prophecies that you won't last anyway to undermine your morale. It won't be long before you will want to avoid the company of smokers for different reasons: the smell of smoke and the stench of stale cigarette butts will offend your re-awakened sense of smell and the smoke itself will irritate your eyes and your respiratory system.

9. If it should happen -- Heaven forbid! -- that, in a moment of temporary insanity, you should have a puff or even a whole cigarette, do not do what you have done in the past -- use that one lapse as an excuse to start smoking again. "That one cigarette" has power over you only if you surrender to it. During the 1972 Olympics, I watched the 10,000-meter race. About half-way through, Lasse Viren, the ace from Finland, collided with another runner and both of them hit the track. Before the 80,000 spectators had fully grasped what had happened, Lasse was up and back in the race. Slowly and steadily he made good lost time, caught up with and passed the rest of the field to win the gold medal and to set a new world

record. A man less determined than he would have used the accident as a legitimate excuse to drop out. In like manner, if you should have the accident of "that one cigarette," the only thing to do is to pick yourself up at once and to carry on as if nothing had happened. Don't listen to temptation whispering, "Poor thing, you've simply taken on too much. Relax for a few days. Permit yourself the small luxury of a few cigarettes You can quit again next week." Don't listen. Surely, if you want to quit, it will be a great deal easier after only one cigarette than it would be a week or two down the road and several packs of cigarettes later.

10. When things get rough, when the agents of temptation have you wholly confused and discouraged, return to this section and re-read it. For, the agents of temptation will keep coming for you for some time. If you chase them out the front door, they will sneak back in by a side door or by a half-open window. It will take constant vigilance not to be taken by surprise. But keep in mind that, with every day you survive as a non-smoker, you will grow stronger and they will grow weaker. Their attacks will become less frequent. Before long you will find that you can go for long periods of time without even remembering that there is such a thing as a cigarette: hours at first, then days, then weeks. Besides, if you refuse to let the agents of temptation draw you into an argument when they come to your door, they will be gone faster than thought, and they may not be back for days. Surely, a few minutes of temptation in the space of several days is something you can live with for a little while. For in due time even this will stop. You will be like one who has never smoked. Every once in a while, when you see others smoke or hear them talk about it, it will come back to you in a flash that, once upon a time, you too were hooked. But now you are free: no more temptation, no more sense of deprivation. Just

the sweet taste of victory. Only those who have gone through it all the way – the getting hooked, the desperate fight for liberation and final victory -- only those understand.

I have been a non-smoker for four decades now. I do not miss smoking at all any more. Every once in a while, when I see others smoke, I remember what it was like to be hooked. There are still moments when I can hardly believe that I really did it, but one deep breath is all it takes to reassure me. The other day I watched a conspicuously rich couple get out of a top-of-the-line Mercedes. I felt a moment's twinge of envy. Then I noticed that she took one last puff of a cigarette she had obviously been smoking in the car and that he was about to light up. How that changed my view of the situation! In that instant I knew that, if they offered me all they owned, perhaps enough money so that I would not have to worry another day in my life, on condition that I start smoking again and continue to smoke till I die, I would tell them without hesitation, "No deal!"

VII

NEW DIRECTIONS

More than forty years have passed since I stopped smoking and more than thirty years since the first edition of this book appeared in Canada.

Much has changed on the tobacco scene since I stopped smoking but much has remained the same. The hazards of smoking,both to the smoker and to the non-smoker exposed to "second-hand" smoke, have been so well documented that not even the most hardened smoker would dare to deny them. Yet hundreds of millions of people the world over still smoke. A former US Surgeon General informed whoever cared to listen that the number of deaths attributable to smoking in the United States each year was greater than the death toll from AIDS, hard drugs, alcohol, fire, murders and car accidents combined. Yet millions of Americans continue to smoke. Smoking, concerned health experts tell us, is probably the most important cause of preventable disease in the world. Tobacco occupies a unique position among consumer goods in that it is the only one that is known to kill if used as intended and can be sold legally to consenting adults. ("The Globe and Mail," Nov. 13, 1991) One Canadian health officer contends that, given our know-ledge of the health consequences of tobacco, no government would allow it if it were to be launched as a new product tomorrow. Yet all governments allow the sale of it TODAY, and a great many governments still permit tobacco companies to use every trick imaginable to recruit new victims for the addiction.

By and large, the number of smokers has gone down in developed countries in the past four decades owing mainly to greater awareness of the hazards of smoking and the pressure interest groups have exerted on governments to take action   Unfortunately tobacco consumption has gone up in developing countries. The main reasons for this are that: 1) tobacco companies have doubled their sales efforts in third-world countries to make up for diminishing sales in developed countries; 2) people in developing countries are less aware of the hazards of smoking; 3) public action groups -- the few that exist -- lack both the funds necessary to educate the public and the political power to pressure governments into action.

Among developed countries fighting tobacco consumption, Canada stands out. Anyone remembering the "bad old days" can't help being aware of some remarkable changes -- changes in the general attitude towards smoking, in smoking behavior, in tobacco consumption and in legislation to curb the activities of the tobacco companies.

When I quit, some forty years ago, smoking was chique in Canada. Today, far from being chique, it is no longer even publicly acceptable. It has, in fact, become chique not to smoke. Non-smokers are no longer willing to put up with being exposed to the risks of second-hand smoke. They get angry when they see someone light up and the smoker himself, sensing the pressure of public disapproval, feels uncomfortable. One smoker told me that it had got so bad -- bad from his point of view -- that, every time he lit up in public, he felt as though he were doing something shameful.

The very meaning of "smoking in public" has narrowed in Canada: it now means little more than smoking out of doors. For there is no more smoking in public buildings such as government offices, universities, schools, department stores or supermarkets. There is no more smoking on city buses, no more smoking on Canadian flights, no mor smoking in restaurants.

Until recently some taverns still allowed patrons to smoke in some closed off restricted areas. I don't know whether this has been outlawed too.

There is no more cigarette advertizing in Canada. By banning tobacco advertizing, the Canadian government has severely limited the opportunities of the tobacco companies to get young people hooked by presenting smoking as part of a glamorous lifestyle. For the edification of those among my readers who think cigarette advertizing has little effect on youngsters taking up smoking, I would like to borrow a few lines from an article in "Arab News" (Dec. 12, 1991) entitled "Cartoon Camel as familiar to kids as Mickey Mouse." Studies done in the US, the article reports, show that Old Joe, a cartoon camel used to promote Camel cigarettes, was as familiar to six-year-olds as Mickey mouse and led to a sharp rise in smoking the Camel brand among teenagers.

Another measure Canada has taken to make it more difficult for youngsters to get hooked is that the sale of tobacco to minors has been prohibited by law in all Canadian provinces, something other countries would do well to copy.

But there is one measure Canada has taken that has done more than all the others combined to discourage smoking – a sharp increase in the cost of tobacco due to higher taxation. When I stopped smoking, four decades ago, a pack of cigarettes cost 40 cents. Anyone could readily afford to smoke then, even teenagers with little spending money. Today a twenty-pack of the pernicious weed costs nearly thirty times as much -- almost twelve Canadian dollars, most of it tax. Twelve dollars would still buy more than a whole carton in most developing countries. I checked in Germany a year ago. There, cigarettes cost about half as much as in Canada.

Steep cigarette prices discourage above all members of the most vulnerable age group, youngsters

aged twelve and up, from experimenting with cigarettes
and so save many of them from becoming hookws..

Tobacco companies put up a stiff fight
against the increase of the tobacco tax in Canada.
Among other things, they succeeded in getting 700,000
smokers to send letters of protest to their government
representatives denouncing the tax hike as undemocratic.
They argued that it was undemocratic because it taxed
unfairly a minority group. Happily the Canadian
government was not moved by the campaign.

Canadian Revenue people are on record as having
said that they increased the tax on tobacco to discourage
its use, especially among the young, and the extra revenue from those that persist in smoking will help defray
the social and medical expenses when the inevitable
happens -- that they become ill and a burden on the state.
TheCanadian Cancer Society, compares the high taxes to
a vaccine.which protects young people against the nicotine addiction. Benoit Bouchard, one-tim minister of
health and welfare, regarded the high taxes on cigarettes
as "preventive medicine." Let other governments follow
suit – make cigarettes so expensive that people will
think twice before they buy a pack.

Thanks to the steps Canada has taken to discourage
the use of tobacco, cigarette consumption has dropped
dramatically over the past three decades and is still
falling. According to a recent report released by tatistics
Canada, Canadians bought only 3.08 billion cigarettes in
June 1991 compared to the 3.93 billion sold in the same
month a year earlier, a whopping 21.6 per cent of a drop.
Cigarette consumption has been going down faster in
Canada than in any other OECD country. Canada has
in fact become a world leader in the fight against tobacco
consumption and experts from dozens of other countries
are studying the measures that have been taken here in
the hope that Canada's success might be repeated in their

own countries.

Much of the credit for the Canadian success story goes to THE NATIONAL PROGRAM TO REDUCE TOBACCO USE, an organization that was established in Canada in the fall of 1985. Its declared purpose is to unite groups in developing an effective, cohesive and comprehensive program to reduce tobacco use. More specifically, the goals of the organization are:

1. to protect the health and rights of the non-smokers
2. to help those who are non-smokers stay smoke-free
3. to encourage and help those who want to quit to do so.

The most important participating members of the organization are Health and Welfare Canada, the Canadian Cancer Society, the Canadian Council on Smoking and Health, the Canadian Public Health Association, the Canadian Medical Association, the Canadian Pharmaceutical Association, the Canadian Lung Association and the Canadian Heart Foundation. The list is impressive. The organization has been concentrating its efforts on

1. sharing information,
2. educational programs for school and community,
3. promotional campaigns,
4. research,
5. community action,
6. promoting appropriate legislation;

and its efforts, as we have seen, have been rewarded with amazing success. But they know that their work is far from over. The success of any anti-smoking campaign ultimately depends on how effective it is in keeping young people from getting started since most new smokers are between 12 and 17 years young. If no more young people start smoking, there will eventually be no more smokers. Tobacco is addictive. Like many anti-smoking campaigners, The Nova Scotia Council of Smoking and Health, is confident that, if we get young people safely through their teens without becoming hooked, they are likely to stay smoke-free for the rest of their lives. They will not thank us, it warns, if we make it too easy for them to become addicts.

Canada's National Program is therefore concentrating its efforts on ways to save the young from becoming addicted. Two new measures it has been proposing are that stores selling cigarettes should be compelled to keep them where they cannot be seen by a casual observer, instead of displaying them in the most prominent places, and that cigarettes should be sold only in generic white packages with black letters spelling out the health warning and the name of the product, nothing else. Research indicates that such packaging would turn teenagers off. The National Program would, moreover, like to see a more effective health warning on cigarette packages.

The other day I went to several of the biggest Jeddah supermarkets for the sole purpose of having a good look at the cigarette displays. The first thing I noticed was that in almost all the stores cigarettes occupy very prominent positions. Single packages fill the racks right beside and above the cash registers. The cartons are parked in shelves which either flank the cash registers or border the approaches to the grocery aisles. Having them placed this way the tobacco companies are sure to catch the attention, not so much of the real nicotine addict -- He would get to the cigarettes if they were kept in an attic five flights of stairs up! -- but of the casual smoker who might otherwise forget to buy cigarettes and so smoke less, and of the teenagers not yet hooked but potential future addicts.

I did more than look at the cigarette displays in general. I picked several individual packs of cigarettes from the racks next to the cash register to have a closer look at them and made some interesting discoveries. I discovered, among other things, that the health message appears only once on each package while the producer's logo appears several times. On one particular package I found the logo seven times -- twice on the surface that faces the smoker when he opens the pack and once each on the remaining five surfaces. I also found that, while the logo comes in different sizes and colors, which virtually leap out at the viewer, the health message is difficult to find and even more difficult to read: the letters that compose it are hard to make out because they are done in colors which offer little contrast to the surface they are printed on; the glare of the cellophane wrapper makes them all but disappear; and, if a smoker does discover the message in spite of all this, he is not likely to be able to read it because the letters are so small that only people with excellent eyesight can make them out.

The long and the short of it is that, in Saudi Arabia, As in virtually all dveloping countries, the health warning on cigarette packages is so ineffective it might as well not be there. The tobacco companies have, while complying with the letter of the law, ignored the spirit of it, which is to warn the potential victim that he is about to buy a killer. I found no health warning on the cigarette cartons though that's where the warning should start. Once a smoker has bought a carton of cigarettes, he is not likely to throw them away. But, if he saw, stamped right on the carton, a health warning in letters or symbols so conspicuous that he could not miss them, his hand extended to grab that carton might well pull back empty. Governments should compel the tobacco companies to produce health warning so prominent that ithey cannot be missed, and those warnings should be stamped, not only on the individual packs of cigarettes but also on the cartons.

The battle against smoking is more than a matter of health. It is a moral issue too. All major religions, foremost among them Islam, forbid their adherents to engage in activities that harm them physically or mentally. Since it has been established beyond a reasonable doubt that smoking is a most serious health hazard, Muslims should abstain from it for moral reasons, if self-interest does not persuade them to do so.

Some Muslim smokers argue that, while the Qu'ran forbids alcohol, it does not forbid smoking. They are the prevaricators, people who twist the truth either to deceive themselves or others. For, though the Qu'ran does not specifically condemn smoking, surely smoking is included in the following summary condemnations of things that harm the body or the mind, or both:

1. And make not your own hands contribute to your destruction. (2:195)
2. Do not kill or destroy yourselves: for verily Allah has been to you most merciful. (4:29)
3. Do not hurt yourselves nor injure others. (Said by the Prophet himself).

The message is clear -- since smoking does harm both to the smoker and to "others," it IS forbidden to Muslims.

If there are any Muslim smokers who are not yet convinced either that smoking does indeed cause harm or that the spirit of Islam forbids smoking, let them buy or borrow a copy of The Growing Threat: Smoking And The Muslim World, published By Abul Qasim Books, Subaiey Center, Box 6156 Jeddah. The half hour it will take them to read this inexpensive little paperback will be time well spent.

Let them, moreover, have a good look at the health

warning on cigarette packages, difficult as it may be to find and to read. There they will learn that "smoking is a major cause of lung cancer and lung diseases and of heart and artery diseases." If the health warning were more detailed, it would tell them that smoking increases the risk of cancer in other areas too, not only in the lungs; e.g., cancers of the mouth, throat, esophagus, pancreas, kidneys and bladder. It would also tell them that the term "lung diseases" can be expanded to include a variety of upper respiratory infections, chronic bronchitis and emphysema; it would tell them that "artery diseases" includes the dreaded stroke; and it would tell them that smoking is a major risk factor in peptic ulcers. If the health warning were to fulfil its purpose, it should carry a warning about the dreadful addictiveness of smoking too.

For the benefit of those who need more convincing, I am going to conclude this chapter by gleaning a few more pieces of information from the wealth of material the Canadian NATIONAL PROGRAM TO REDUCE TOBACCO USE has supplied – information which, though it reflects causes and effects in Canada, is indeed applicable anywhere.

The real drug problem of Canada, says Dr. Mark Taylor of the Nova Scotia Council on Smoking and Health, is not illegal drugs but nicotine, the legal drug. About 400 deaths occur annually from the use of illegal drugs while tobacco, the legal drug, kills more than 38,000 a year. Alcohol, the only other drug that belongs in the same league as tobacco, kills a mere 20% of that, or about 7,000.

A study by Canada's Department of Health and Welfare reports that in 1985 there were 11,400 lung cancer deaths in Canada, 80% of them directly attributable to smoking. Some 330 of these lung cancer deaths occurred in non-smokers as a result of exposure to second-hand smoking. Non-smokers are at risk from all the other health problems associated with smoking too. For children, the risk begins before birth. Health and Welfare Canada reports that active smoking by pregnant women is linked to miscarriage and stillbirth. In live births, it is linked to lower fetal birth weight and growth retardation. Children of parents who smoke have a higher incidence of respiratory problems than children who grow up in smokeless homes. If they suffer from asthma, they often have their condition aggravated by involuntary smoking.

According to another study by Health and Welfare Canada, smoking was responsible for one in five deaths in Canada in 1989.... Can there be people, I wonder, who are so foolish as to think that smoking kills only Canadians but spares other nationalities? If not, how can they persist in smoking?

I have a dream that other countries will, encouraged by the example of Canada, also declare war on what Dr. Taylor calls the death industry. I have a dream that this little book of mine may help some of the millions of smokers struggling to extricate themselves from the tentacles of the monster. I have a dream that I will live to see the day when selling tobacco will be viewed as a crime anywhere in the world, much as selling hard drugs is now.

APPENDIX A

What to Eat

The intent of the nutritional program is that you should eat yourself into a state of health so nearly perfect that, as much as that's possible, all hidden hungers resulting from nutritional deficiencies will be stilled and all biochemical imbalances will be corrected. For, any such deficiencies or imbalances can translate themselves into cravings, your body's signals that something is missing. Unfortunately, your body has no wy of letting you know specifically what's missing. The cravings it sends you remain, for the most part, vague and indiscriminate. They are as likely to push you towards sugar, caffeine or NICOTINE as they are to push you towards food that could supply what's missing.

To remedy the hidden deficiencies or imbalances in the ecology of your body, all you need to do is eat a reasonably well balanced diet of natural food, unrefined and processed no more than necessary to render it edible. Your body will do the rest. Among other things, this means hands off "edible petroleum products"; it means potatoes baked in their skins, not potato chips; it means eating a hole apple or a whole orange rather than drinking apple or orange juice; it means a whole-wheat cereal rather than puffed wheat or corn flakes, etc. Late research, by the way, outlaws wheat altogether because of the glutin it contains. Whole rye, rolled oats and unrefined barley are eligible grains.

Assemble your diet of natural, unrefined and unprocessed foods from among the following:

Fruit and vegetalbes: Eat what is in season, preferably fresh and raw. In Canadian latitudes, there is not much to choose from during the winter months. Oranges, apples, bananas, grapes and cantaloupes -- you quickly run out of things that are affordable during the cold part of the year. Go easy on the dried varieties of fruit such as raisins, figs, dates, etc. Too much of them can upset your sugar metabolism. Have fruit at your coffee break,morning and afternoon. If only canned fruit is available, go for fruit canned without sugar. Hands off canned fruit that is packed in sticky-sweet sugar syrup. Try a home-made fruit salad with a bit of home-made yogurt. Delicious! Vegetables: Again, eat whatever happens to be in season and therefore cheapest. Eat as many of your vegetables raw as possible. However, while most vegetables are best eaten raw,some of them such as carrots, turnips and squash yield more of their nutritional goodness if they are parboiled. The cellulose of their cell walls is so tough that the human digestive machinery succeeds only partly in breaking it down. Cooking helps, but do not overcook and do not throw away the water in which you cook your vegetables. Try this for a delicious salad:

2 to 3 sticks of celery
1 green pepper
1/2 avocado   chop
1 medium onion
1/2 head of lettuce

1/2 cucumber   grate
1 to 2 carrots

3 T of apple cider vinegar
3 T of cold-pressed oil
2 T of soy sauce
a sprinkle of curry

Try adding a few crumbs of Danish Blue, or crumble a

hard-boiled egg into your salad. I frequently have this sort of salad for breakfast.

Seeds and Cereals: Nature packs plenty of nutritional punch into seeds to ensure germination and growth. Seeds include not only things like sunflower seeds and sesame seeds; they also include peas and beans and nuts and grains. Take some sunflower seeds or some nuts (unsalted, unroasted) with you, wherever you go, for quick and highly nutritious snacks. Grind some nuts in your coffee grinder to sprinkle on fruit salads or on your yogurt. Use unrefined "seeds" for breakfast cereals: delicious mixtures of various types of grain, nuts and bits of dried fruit are available as "granola" at natural food outlets. Buy your rolled oats at the natural food outlet too; for what you find at the supermarket is usually the instant or the semi-instant variety. Get some of your seeds in the form of delicious whole-grain pumpernickle.

Cheeses: Hands off the processed cheeses -- the stuff that spreads, like the cheese spreads in glass jars or in cellophane casings. Most natural food outlets and, of course, delicatessens offer a wonderful selection of non-processed cheeses. Sample them all to begin with and determine your favorites. Mine are cheddar, anfleur, oka, brie, gouda and tilsit. In my area, Costco offers faraway the best eelection of cheeses and the best prices.

Milk: As I said before, don't consider milk a drink; consider it a food. A glass of milk is fine for a snack between meals but don't use milk to wash down your food with at meals.Meat: I won't try to settle the argument whether a vegetarian diet is better than a diet that includes meat though privately I believe that vege-tarians by and large enjoy above average health and have a higher life expectancy than meat eaters. I agree with those who hold that, while a vegetarian diet is excellent for many people, not everyone could or would want to live on it permanently. Ultimately only you yourself can tell what's best for you. If you cannot or will not live without meat, at least consider reducing your meat intake. You don't need meat to be healthy. You certainly don't need meat with every meal. Eat more fish and foul than beef or mutton; if you must have beef or mutton, eat only lean cuts, and eat organ meats -- liver, heart, kidney, etc. Whether fish or foul, beef or mutton, have your meats boiled (in stews), broiled or roasted rather than fried. And go easy on canned fish like tuna, salmon or sardines:they contain too much salt. Hands off canned meats, though; most of them have sugar added and contain undesirable additives. Hands off processed meats in general. The only processing you should settle for is the processing that happens in your own kitchen.

A list of things to eat would be criminally incomplete if it did not contain some of the special foods like wheat germ, brewer's yeast, sprouted seeds, yogurt, etc. These are not new-fangled fad foods. They are as old as human memory. It is only in humanity's latest generation or two that they have become the forgotten foods, chiefly thanks to the corporate food processors who try to steer us in the direction of processed food. If you'd like to know just what makes these foods so special, read up on them in "Feel Like A Million" or in "Know Your Nutrition." I'll limit myself to listing them and to pointing out how much to take and what to do with them.

Liver: A nutritional power house. Whether you are a carnivore or a vegetarian, you should eat liver now and then, perhaps as often as once a week. It will yield big health dividends.

Wheat Germ: Another power house of good nutrition.

Though it is the most valuable part of the wheat kernel, it is removed in the milling process and fed to animals. Human beings are treated to the almost empty calories of the refined white flour. Wheat germ can be added to cereals, to whole-grain baking done at home, to fruit salads. It is delicious with a mashed banana and some milk. The gluten content of wheat germ is naglibible.

Brewer's Yeast: Though one of the most valuable foods, I almost hesitate to include it in my list of special foods; for most people don't find it palatable, at least not until they acquire a taste for it. Try taking it in juice -- orange, apple, tomato – and shake or blend it well so that no lumps remain. Start off with a teaspoonful a day. Gradually work your way up to at least a tablespoon a day. Don't panic if, for a few days, perhaps for a week or two after you start taking brewer's yeast, you develop strange abdominal rumblings. They do not mean that brewer's yeast does not agree with you; on the contrary, they are a sign that you need it very much. You see, brewer's yeast is chock-full of B-vitamins, a deficiency of which often results in intestinal sluggishness. With the sudden influx of the B's in brewer's yeast, the lower half of your digestive machinery wakes to new life, and as it gets into high gear, these rumblings develop. Don't worry about them. They will disappear in time. By the way, liver and wheat germ, if suddenly introduced into a diet that has been deficient in the B's, can cause some abdominal rumblings too; for they are close rivals of brewer's yeast in being among the best dietary sources of the B-Vitamins.

Bran: If you take one to three tablespoons of bran daily, you can say good-bye to laxatives forever. There is one minor problem though: this best dietary source of fiber, which has virtually no taste of its own, does not go down very well because of is texture. It's almost impossible to eat it by itself because it does not yield to chewing. I know of people who take it in tomato juice. You can add some to your cereal or to your to-be-baked-at-home bread. I mix mine with ground nuts – two parts of nuts to one part of bran -- and soak the mixture in milk or water for some 15 minutes. When I eat it, I hardly become aware that there is bran in it.

Lecithin: Nutrition experts in whom I have confidence tell me that lecithin helps to keep cholesterol in my blood honest and thus prevents it from solidifying and clogging my arteries. It seems the answer to the cholesterol problem is not so much trying to avoid such good foods as eggs, nuts and butter but to eat some lecithin. It comes in granules or in easy-to-take capsules. The latter are relatively expensive; granules, on the other hand, though much cheaper, are difficult to take for some people. I for one like both the taste and the texture of lecithin, and I take it straight from the spoon. If you cannot do that, try taking it in tomato juice. If you cannot get it down any other way, by all means get yourself some capsules.

Sprouts: Another food with lots of nutritional punch. Before you start sprouting your own seeds, buy some ready-to-eat sprouts at a natural food outlet or at a supermarket. You'll find bean sprouts in the vegetable section of many a supermarket. If you like them, grow your own. The chapter "Vitamin-Rich Sprouts" in Feel Like A Million offers simple and effective directions how to sprout seeds. You can eat your sprouts by them-selves, or you can add them to salads or to vegetable stews. Cook your stew first. When it is almost done, add the sprouts and simmer for a few more minutes. If you cooked them more, much of their nutritional goodness would be lost.

Cold-pressed oils: "Cold-pressed" means extracted by a process of mechanical pressing, without the use of heat, without the use of chemicals. Some oil merchants have presses to extract oil from your choice of seeds while you wait. That's the best kind of cold-pressed oil. But don't buy big quantities of it. Buy no more than you can use in the space of a month or two. And keep it in a cool dark place at home. Olive oil that's labelled "extra virgin" is reliably cold-pressed too. It is important that you get some cold-pressed oil frequently, perhaps half a tablespoon to a tablespoon a day. Safflower oil, sesame seed oil, peanut oil, sunflower oil, olive oil -- any of these will do as long as they are cold-pressed. Most of the oils you find in the supermarkets are not cold-pressed. They are oils extracted by a process that involves heating and the addition of chemicals. Besides, most of them contain preservatives to keep them from spoiling. Cold-pressed oils spoil rather quickly after the bottles containing them have been opened. So keep your cold-pressed oils in the fridge. You can add some cold-pressed oil to your salads. If you put a tablespoon of it in your hot cereal, you won't even notice it. Use some in your baking.

Yogurt: Hands off the flavored varieties of yogurt. They contain sugar and other additives. If you cannot get used to plain yogurt, create your own flavored varieties. Mashed bananas, strawberries or peaches combine deliciously with plain yogurt. And consider making your own yogurt. It is cheaper, it tastes better and it is better for you than the yogurts you buy.

No need to buy a yogurt maker; you don't need one to make yogurt. Here is my own no-nonsense method of making yogurt, the result of much trial and error. I have been making my own yogurt for some 40 years. Would not touch any of the commencial yogurts. Most of them have been pasteurized to increase the shelf life of the product but pasteurizing destroys the most valuable part of yogurt – the yogurt bacteria, which are virtually identical with healthy body flroa.

I usually use 10 /% cream. You can make yogurt

with regular whole milk but it does not thicken properly. It would still make good yogurt even it it doesn thicken. You can reeconstitute powdered milk in luke-warm water. in the blender. Add about 2 tablespoons of "starter" to a blender bowl. The starter is merely plain yogurt. The first time you have to "import" a starter. Get a yogurt culture from a health food store. Failing that, look for a commercial yogurt that has not been pasteurized. A yogurt that has been pasteurized won't work as a starter because pasteurizing kills the bacterial culture that transforms milk into yogurt. But once you have your own yogurt, all you have to do is save a spoonful or two of it from one batch to the next to use as a starter.

Put the milk cum starter in a bowl, cover it and leave it in a warm place. While "incubating," its temperature should be somewhere between 80o F (27o C) and body temperature. If it is too cold, it won't "hatch"; if too hot, the starter dies and it won't "hatch" either. In either case you will end up with spoiled milk rather than yogurt. If conditions are right, it will make itself in 4 to 6 hours. Experiment with a few small batches first. When you have the hang of it, you can make big batches.

Having told you in broad terms what to eat, I should tell you briefly what to drink. After all, I have pronounced a ban on coffee, tea (a cup of weak tea, by the way, as a treat now and then is all right), and soft drinks. What is there left to drink?

There are still many things to choose from. But, before I point them out to you, let me tell you that, if you adopt the dietary changes recommended in Chapter IV, you will need much less of anything to drink than you used to; for, a diet that consists largely of natural foods, including significant quantities of raw fruit and vegetables, will give you almost allyou need of fluids. A reduced salt intake, moreover, will mean lower fluid requirements. But you will get thirsty, especially when you exercise or when you spend much time al fresco and you \will want something to drink. When you do, choose from among the following:

Water. Depending on where you live, especially if you live in a big city, where tap water may be laced with chlorine and chances are that it may contain fluoride and traces of other pollutants, it may be advisable for you to buy bottled water for your drinking purposes. But even if the water from your tap is not what it should be, it is nevertheless preferable to water that has been further corrupted by the addition of a variety of substances detrimental to health -- coffee, sugar and chemicals as in soft drinks, artificial fruit flavors in "fruit drinks." Yes, from a health point of view, soft drinks are polluted water. They may not contain bacteria or traces of pesticides but they containsubstances that do you harm.
 I like a glass of mineral water now and then. My favorite brand is Apollinaris, imported from Germany. However, at more than two dollars a bottle it is not something I buy every day.
Fruit juices. Only genuine juices, none of the fruit drinks. While you are getting ready to quit, and for some time after, you should go easy even on genuine fruit juices; for they too can disturb your sugar metabolism. After all, a fruit juice is a processed food. When it enters your digestive system, very little further "processing" is necessary for what there is of sugar to be absorbed into your blood stream. If you drink more than a very few ounces of all but the sourest juices, your blood stream can be so flooded with glucose that your pancreas is spooked into a fit of hyperactivity that can trigger hypoglycemia. So drink only small quantities of fruit juice. Take it as a "desert" rather than as a thirst quencher. If you are

thirsty and you won't settle for water, dilute your juices --
one part of juice to two parts of water -- to get a delicious thirst quencher, the sugar content of which is low
enough not to upset your blood sugar metabolism or your
calorie count.

Surrogate coffee. Natural food outlets sell various
brands of herbal coffee. Sample them. You will be
surprised how much like real coffee they taste. And they
are nutritionally safe, their principal ingredients being
ground roasted wheat or barley and chicory root. Try a
cup of postum. If you can't find any of them in your
neighborhood stores, make your own. Nothing to it.
Just roast some wheat or barley, grind it in your coffee
grinder or your blender and treat it as you would ground
coffee beans.

Herbal teas. Herbal teas are very popular in much of
Europe, especially in Germany and in Switzerland. In
North America, many people recoil as before something
unclean when I suggest that they drink herbal teas
instead of regular tea. They forget that regular tea is
itself a herbal tea. The important difference between
regular tea and other herbal teas is that the former,
much like coffee, is a stimulant -- it gives you a "lift."
But that is precisely the effect you want to avoid while
getting ready to quit smoking and for some time
afterwards. Herbal teas are safe. You find them at
natural food outlets and at delicatessens. Most supermarkets carry at least mint and camomile. My favorites
are spearmint, peppermint, rose hip, elderflower and
lemon grass. Discover your own favorites. You can have
them hot or cold. During the summer months, I always
have a pitcher of herbal tea in the fridge. Iced mint tea
with a few drops of lemon juice is a delicious summer
drink. **Non-alcoholic beer**. Made essentially from the
same ingredients as real beer, it tastes deceptively like
real beer. In Germany and in Switzerland it has long

been the beer of children and of pregnant women.

A word or two about supplements before I conclude this section. If circumstances were ideal -- if we had access to clean, mineral-rich water at all time; if our food were grown organically on balanced soils; if our diets were truly balanced diets of natural foods; if we, and our parents, had always abstained from such noxious substances as coffee, tea, refined sugar and nicotine; if we had always had sufficient exercise -- there would probably be no need for supplements. However, circumstances being less than ideal for us, most of us could benefit from some supplementation. At the same time, individual needs vary so greatly that it is really impossible to make any generally valid ecommendations. The only thing to do in the circumstances is to give you a basic list of those supplements which most people engaged in a program of rebuilding health could benefit from.

Vitamins A and D. They usually come together in capsules of 5,000 I(nternational) U(nits) of A and 400 mcg of D. Take one or two a day. I recomment some extra Vitamin D, especially during the winter months, when most mid-latitude people are deficient in Vitamin D because they lack exposure to the sun.

Vitamin D is a much better protection against the flu than the flu shot. Why do we have flu epidemics in winter but not in summer? You'll do yourself a big favor if you search for and read "Just One Pill Away" to learn that Vitamin D – D3, by the way, not the syntheic D2 – does much more than protect you against the flu and other respiratory infections; that, among other things, it reduces the incidence of a variety of cancers (prostate, breast, ovary, colon among them), of heart attacks, of multiple sxlerosis and more. I recommend 5,000 mcg from October to April and, depending on the amount of sun exposure, +/- 2000 mcg from May to September.

Though I am past 80 and, though I have never had a flu shot --- they'd have to tie me down to get the shot into me – I am no more afraid of getting the flu than I am of being struck by lightning. Right now, Alberta is setting up new clinics to administer the flu shot, but not a whisper about Vitamin 3, the sunshine vitamin, which is our best and out cheapest protector against the flu. This is, no doubt the doing of Big Pharma. It will collect billionas without doing any good. If you want to be protected against the annual flu epidemic, take at least 5000 IU of D3 a day but stay away from the flu shot.

The B-vitamins. If you eat the B-rich foods -- wheat germ,brewer's yeast, liver -- you need not worry about your intake of the B's. Otherwise get yourself a B-complex suppl ement that contains all the B's, all eleven of them. (B1, B2, B3, B5, B6, B12, Biotin, Choline, Inositoal, Pantothenic Acid and Folic Acid).

Vitamin C. 1,000 to 2,000 mg a day, divided into four or five smaller doses and taken through the day.

Vitamin E. 200 to 400 IU a day. If you suffer from high blood pressure or a rheumatic heart condition, consult a doctor who is knowledgeable about Vitamin E or read what Linda Clark has to say about it. (Know Your Nutrition, p. 48). At any rate, start at low doses – 100 mcg a day and gradually – over a few months – work up to 400 mcg a day. Incidentally, with Vitamin E, mcg is equivalent to International Unites.

Calcium and magnesium. Take one or two tablets of dolomite a day. Dolomite supplies the two minerals in the right proportion. If you consume alcohol, you had better take some extra Magnesium.

APPENDIX B

More About Exercise

Each of Dr. Cooper's books contains a set of tables from which you can determine how much time you must invest in the exercise of your choice in order to become or to remain fit. If, for instance, walking is your choice, you must do 4 miles a day in from one hour to 80 minutes 4 times a week. If you are a super walker who can do 4 miles in less than 58 minutes, you need to go walking only 3 days a week. If it's jogging, 1.5 miles in less than 15 minutes five times a week is enough. If you'd rather play squash, handball or basketball, you need 40 minutes 5 times a week. Dr. Cooper offers detailed charts for many more types of exercise such as bad-minton, golf, skating, tennis, etc. In all, you will find a choice of some 20 different types of exercise in his books, among which there must be at least one to tempt you.

The exercise of my choice is running. I do other things occasionally: I go swimming or cycling; I go for long walks now and then; once in a while I play a vigorous game of table tennis. But I consider these things entertainment rather than exercise. An evening of ping-pong is for me what an evening at the tavern is for my neighbor. No, for me exercise is running.

When I first started to jog -- jog or run, I use the terms interchangeably -- some forty years ago, I was desperately out of shape and about 40 pounds too heavy. The first few weeks of it were sheer torture, and it took all I had of self-discipline to keep going. To make matters worse, I did what many sudden converts do -- I tried for too much too fast and I developed all sorts of achea and pains. For some time my feet were so sore in the morning that I had to work them gingerly for several minutes before I could walknormally. My whole body was an assortment of aches and pains, the wages of my impatience. If I had to do it again, I'd be much easier on myself and avoid most of the misery. However, I was fortunate in that most of the pains subsided after a couple of months. Though I still smoked then, my breathing improved. Very gradually running ceased to be a chore and it started to be fun.

Here is how I went about breaking myself in: I'd jog gently till out of breath -- 100 yards or less would easily accomplish that -- then I'd slow to a walk till my breathing was back to normal. Back to jogging till out of breath again, slow to a walk, etc. I'd keep this up for about 15 minutes. Gradually the jogging intervals grew longer and the walking intervals grew shorter. I don't remember how long it took before I could run the whole 15 minutes without having to slow to a walk, but I remember how proud I felt and how buoyed with hope I was that day. I may not have covered much more than a mile in those 15 minutes, but I knew that I had come a long way. Now I run five kilometers a day five times a week and I do one longer run on weekends -- 10 km, 15 km, and now and then I tackle 20 km.

Running has long ceased to be a chore. If it had continued to be a chore, I would not have kept it up for four decades. Running is something I look forward to because it makes me feel good physically and mentally. The few days when I don't get to run I don't feel right.

Let me tell you why, though I have sampled other kinds of exercise, I have singled out and stuck to running. Perhaps the most important reason is that running gives me more training value in less time than any other form of aerobic exercise readily available to me. Compare the amount of time one has to invest in each of the following activities in order to obtain what Dr. Cooper considers the basic minimum of exercise value:

Exercise	Total time per week
Running	40 minutes
Rope skipping	an hour and three-quarters
Swimming	2 hours or more
Basketball	3 hours or more
Walking	2 to 5 hours

Don't get me wrong. I am not one to skimp on my time for exercise. I just like the fact that running gives me more training value per time unit than practically any other form of aerobic exercise readily available to me.

Another advantage of running is that I need not buy any expensive equipment. The price of a good pair of running shoes -- $ 40 to $ 100 -- is all I need to invest. And I need not waste time getting to and from my theater of action. I can step into it from my front porch, and I can time my run so that the end of it gets me back to my point of departure.

I can run at any time -- morning, afternoon or night. No need to synchronize my effort with the opening hours of the swimming pool or the gym; no need to wait for partners or team-mates. The only thing that interferes with my running now and then is really bad weather. But there are not many days in a Canadian year which are so totally bad from morning till night that I cannot get half an hour of running in some time. And if it storms without intermission from one end of the day to he other, I put in a day of rest. Otherwise, I let neither the cold of Canadian winters nor the heat of tropical hot seasons interfere with my running.

There is something else about running that appeals to me. It gives me a chance to do some very special sight-seeing. I like to watch the world come alive when I run in the morning. I hardly ever run the same route twice. If I run in daylight, I run whichever way "the wind blows me," always curious what will meet my eyes around the next corner. Now and then a passing car honks its horn at me -- friends or acquaintances trying to catch my attention. During a decade of teaching at one of the largest schools in Eastern Canada, I got to know hundreds students.They are grown people now, but many of them remember me; and, no matter where I run, I am as likely as not to get waved or honked at by one of them. But I like running at night too, especially when the moon is out to put its fairy-tale hue of silver over all things.

So, go buy yourself one of Dr. Cooper's books and browse through it. Get yourself started on an aerobics program of your own. Age is no barrier. You can do it if you are in the tenth decade of life. The benefits won't be long in coming: an improved cardiovascular system will result in better circulation; in all probability your blood pressure will go down; you will lose weight; you will bid farewell to problems like constipation and insomnia; you will feel more vigorous and younger than you have felt in years, and you will look younger too; and, perhaps most important of all, aerobic exercise will be one of your staunchest allies in your fight against smoking. Be confident. I have known scores of smokers who, after they had been engaged in their form of aerobic exercise for a while, gave up smoking. It happens almost inevitably; for aerobic exercise and smoking don't go together. In time, you give up one or the other.

THE END

AFTERWORD

Writing this book has been fun, chiefly because it has been a constant reminder that I am a non-smoker. The thought that it may help some of the millions of people still hooked on nicotine to get themselves unhooked has been exciting too. The approach it advocates works. It worked for me, and it has worked for a number of veteran smokers who had not been able to quit any other way. I hope it will work for you.

If it does, let me know. Please write to me. Tell me what you think of the book. If you have any suggestions for improving it, let me know. I may some day decide to rewrite it. If I do, I'll be glad to incorporate your suggestions.

Address all correspondence to:

Ambros Prechtl, ND PhD
201-26 Alton Drive
Halifax, NS B3N 1L9 Canada
902-477-8221

BIBLIOGRAPHY

1.   Abrahamson, E.B. and Prezet, A.W. BODY
      MIND AND SUGAR. Pyramid Books, New.
      York, 1973

2.   Airola, Paavo, Ph.D. ARE YOU CONFUSED?
      Health Plus Publishers, Phoenix, Arizona, 1977.

3.   Atkins, M.D. DR. ATKINS DIET REVO-
      LUTION. Bantam Book, New York, 1973.

4.   Bieler, Henry G. FOOD IS YOUR BEST
      MEDICINE. Vintage Books, New York, 1973.

5.   Bloomfield, H.H., M.D., et. al. TM: DISCOVER-
      ING INNER   ENERGY AND OVERCOMING
      STRESS. Dell Publishing Cp/. New York, 1975.

6.   Brean, Herbert. HOW TO STOP SMOKING.
      Pocket Books,   New York, 1976.

7.   Caldwell, Ernest. HOW YOU CAN STOP
      SMOKING   PERMANENTLY. Wilshire Book
      Company, 1975.

8.   Clark, Linda. KNOW YOUR NUTRITION.
      Keats Publishing, New Canaan, Connecticut,
1973.

9.   Cooper, Kenneth H., M.D. AEROBICS. Bantam
      Books, New York, 1972.

10.   Cooper, Mildred and Cooper, Kenneth H., M.D.
      AEROBICS   FOR WOMEN. Bantam Books, New

York, 1972.

11. Cott, Allan, M.D. FASTING AS A WAY OF
    LIFE. Bantam Books, New York, 1977.

12. Cott, Allan, M.D. FASTING: THE ULTIMATE
    DIET. Bantam Books, New York, 1975.

13. Dufty, William. SUGAR BLUES. Warner
    Books, New York, 1975.

14. Dunn Trop, Jack. PLEASE DON'T SMOKE IN
    OUR HOUSE. Natural Hygiene Press,
    Chicago, 1976.

15. Elwood, Catharyn. FEEL LIKE A MILLION.
    Pocket Books, New York, 1972.

16. Fredericks, Carlton, Ph.D. and Goodman
    Herman, M.D. LOW BLOOD SUGAR AND
    YOU. Constellation International,
    New York, 1973.

17. Health and Welfare Canada. HOW WE QUIT
    SMOKING. Information Canada.

18. Hittleman, Richard. YOGA: 28 DAY EXERCISE
    PLAN. Workman Publishing Company, New
    York, 1969.

19. LeShan, Lawrence. HOW TO MEDITATE.
    Bantam Books, New York, 1975.

20. Moore Lappé, Frances. DIET FOR A SMALL
    PLANET. Ballantine Books, New York, 1972.

21. Morehouse, Lawrence E., Ph.D. TOTAL FITNESS. Simon and Schuster, New York, 1975.

22. Robin, Anthony. UNLIMITED POWER. Ballantine, 1986.

23. Shelton, Herbert M. FASTING CAN SAVE YOUR LIFE. Hygiene Press, Chicago, 1967.

24. Taha Ahmed. THE GROWING THREAT: SMOKING AND THE MUSLIM WORLD. Abul Qasim Bookstore, Jeddah, 1989.

25. Tozer, Eliot. THE THINKING MAN'S GUIDE TO QUITTING CIGARETTES. Award Books, New York, 1971.

26. Watts, Allan. MEDITATION. Celestial Arts, 231 Adrian Road, Millbrae, California, 1974.

27. Webb, Audry T. SLIMMING WITH YOGA. Simon and Schuster, New York, 1970.

28. Williams, Roger, Ph.D. NUTRTITION AGAINST DISEASE. Bantam Books, New York, 1973.